Perspectives on

HEALTH
EQUITY

& Social Determinants of Health

Kimber Bogard, Velma McBride Murry,
Charlee Alexander, Editors

A Special Publication of the

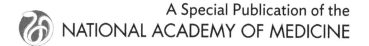 NATIONAL ACADEMY OF MEDICINE

NATIONAL ACADEMY OF MEDICINE • 500 FIFTH STREET, NW • WASHINGTON, DC 20001

NOTICE: This publication has been reviewed according to procedures approved by a National Academy of Medicine (NAM) report review process. Publication signifies that it is judged a competent and useful contribution worthy of public consideration, but does not imply endorsement of conclusions and recommendations by the NAM. The views presented in this publication are those of individual authors and do not represent formal consensus positions of the NAM; the National Academies of Sciences, Engineering, and Medicine; or the authors' organizations.

Support for this activity was provided by the NAM's Kellogg Health of the Public Fund.

Library of Congress Cataloging-in-Publication Data

Names: Bogard, Kimber, editor. | Murry, Velma McBride, editor. | Alexander, Charlee M., editor. | National Academy of Medicine (U.S.), issuing body
Title: Perspectives on health equity and social determinants of health / Kimber Bogard, Velma McBride Murry, and Charlee Alexander, editors.
Description: Washington, DC : National Academy of Medicine, [2017]
Identifiers: LCCN 2017036543 (print) | LCCN 2017036909 (ebook) | ISBN 9781947103030 (Ebook) | ISBN 9781947103023 (pbk.)
Subjects: | MESH: Social Determinants of Health | Health Equity | United States
Classification: LCC RA445 (ebook) | LCC RA445 (print) | NLM WA 30 | DDC 362.10973--dc23
LC record available at https://lccn.loc.gov/2017036543

Suggested citation: Bogard, K., V. Murry, and C. Alexander, eds. 2017. *Perspectives on health equity and social determinants of health.* Washington, DC: National Academy of Medicine.

"Knowing is not enough; we must apply.
Willing is not enough; we must do."

—Goethe

LEADERSHIP
INNOVATION
IMPACT

for a healthier future

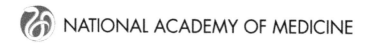 NATIONAL ACADEMY OF MEDICINE

ABOUT THE NATIONAL ACADEMY OF MEDICINE

The **National Academy of Medicine** is one of three Academies constituting the National Academies of Sciences, Engineering, and Medicine (the National Academies). The National Academies provide independent, objective analysis and advice to the nation and conduct other activities to solve complex problems and inform public policy decisions. The National Academies also encourage education and research, recognize outstanding contributions to knowledge, and increase public understanding in matters of science, engineering, and medicine.

The **National Academy of Sciences** was established in 1863 by an Act of Congress, signed by President Lincoln, as a private, nongovernmental institution to advise the nation on issues related to science and technology. Members are elected by their peers for outstanding contributions to research. Dr. Marcia McNutt is president.

The **National Academy of Engineering** was established in 1964 under the charter of the National Academy of Sciences to bring the practices of engineering to advising the nation. Members are elected by their peers for extraordinary contributions to engineering. Dr. C. D. Mote, Jr., is president.

The **National Academy of Medicine** (formerly the Institute of Medicine) was established in 1970 under the charter of the National Academy of Sciences to advise the nation on issues of health, medical care, and biomedical science and technology. Members are elected by their peers for distinguished contributions to medicine and health. Dr. Victor J. Dzau is president.

Learn more about the National Academy of Medicine at NAM.edu.

AUTHORS

CARL C. BELL, MD, Jackson Park Hospital and Windsor University

PATRICK H. DELEON, PHD, MPH, JD, Uniformed Services University of the Health Sciences

ANGELA DIAZ, MD, Phd, MPH, Icahn School of Medicine, Mount Sinai

KAREN E. DILL-SHACKLEFORD, Phd, Fielding Graduate University

LAWRENCE M. DRAKE II, Phd, MA, MBA, LEAD Program

VIVIAN L. GADSDEN, Edd, University of Pennsylvania

HELENE GAYLE, MD, MPH, Chicago Community Trust

WALTER S. GILLIAM, Phd, Yale School of Medicine

COTI-LYNNE PUAMANA HAIA, JD, Office of Hawaiian Affairs

JEFF HUTCHINSON, MD, FAAP, Uniformed Services University of the Health Sciences

JOSEPH KEAWE'AIMOKU KAHOLOKULA, Phd, University of Hawai'i

TRACEY PÉREZ KOEHLMOOS, Phd, MHA, Marine Corps

RICHARD M. LERNER, Phd, Tufts University

NANCY LÓPEZ, Phd, University of New Mexico

RAQUEL MACK, MS, Uniformed Services University of the Health Sciences

JIM MARKS, MD, MPH, Robert Wood Johnson Foundation

SHANTEL E. MEEK, Phd, Administration for Children and Families

NOREEN MOKUAU, DSW, University of Hawai'i

VELMA MCBRIDE MURRY, Phd, Vanderbilt University

KEN PEAKE, DSW, Mount Sinai Adolescent Health Center and Icahn School of Medicine at Mount Sinai

DWAYNE PROCTOR, Phd, Robert Wood Johnson Foundation

SRIVIDYA RAMASUBRAMANIAN, Phd, MA, Texas A&M University

ROBERT SEIDEL, MLA, McDaniel College

SADÉ SOARES, Uniformed Services University of the Health Sciences

PATRICK H. TOLAN, Phd, University of Virginia

SHARON TOOMER, BlackandBrownNews.com

★Affiliations current as of December 2017

JOANN U. TSARK, MPH, University of Hawai'i, Native Hawaiian Board of Health, and Native Hawaiian Cancer Network
ALFORD A. YOUNG JR., PhD, University of Michigan

NAM Staff

KIMBER BOGARD, PhD, Senior Officer
CHARLEE ALEXANDER, Program Officer
LAURA DeSTEFANO, Director of Communications
KYRA E. CAPPELUCCI, Communications Specialist
MOLLY DOYLE, Communications Specialist

REVIEWERS

The papers in this volume were reviewed in draft form by individuals chosen for their diverse perspectives and technical expertise, in accordance with review procedures approved by the National Academy of Medicine. We wish to thank the following individuals for their review of the papers in this volume:

CLARA L. ADAMS-ENDER, United States Army Nurse Corps *(retired)*
DAVID A. BRENT, MD, University of Pittsburgh
DAVID V. B. BRITT, MPA, Sesame Workshop *(retired)*
HERNAN CARVENTE, BS, Youth First
MARK E. COURTNEY, Phd, University of Chicago
ELENA FUENTES-AFFLICK, MD, MPH, University of California, San Francisco
AMY LEFFLER, Phd, MSW, U.S. Department of Justice
HARRY J. HOLZER, Phd, Georgetown University
LARKE N. HUANG, Phd, Substance Abuse and Mental Health Services Administration
JEFF HUTCHINSON, MD, Uniformed Services University of the Health Sciences
ANN S. MASTEN, Phd, University of Minnesota
CHRISTINE RAMEY, MBA, BSN, RN, Health Resources and Services Administration
MARTÍN J. SEPÚLVADA, MD, MPH, Fellow, IBM
MELISSA A. SIMON, MD, Northwestern University Feinberg School of Medicine
BELINDA E. SIMS, Phd, National Institute on Drug Abuse
MILDRED THOMPSON, MSW, PolicyLink Center for Health Equity and Place *(retired)*

Although the reviewers listed above provided many constructive comments and suggestions, they were not asked to endorse the content of the papers, nor did they see the final drafts before publication. Review of these papers was overseen by **Kimber Bogard, PhD,** Senior Officer for Planning and Advancement and Managing Officer, Culture of Health Program, NAM. Responsibility for the final content of these papers rests entirely with the authors and the NAM.

PREFACE

On May 11, 2015, the Board on Children, Youth, and Families of the National Academies of Sciences, Engineering, and Medicine (the National Academies), held a public meeting to discuss the social determinants of health inequities and social injustice using a social justice lens. The meeting, "Armchair Discussions of Social Justice and Equity across the Life Course," engaged academicians, policy makers, policy implementers, community service providers, and community representatives who work with vulnerable populations to achieve four objectives: (1) address the laws, policies, and leadership needed to ensure social justice and health equity for children, youth, and families; (2) highlight "institutions" such as parenting, the juvenile justice system, the foster care system, the school system, and the ways these institutions protect the development of children and youth in the context of social justice and health equity; (3) focus on health disparities resulting from discriminatory practices and policies, and missed opportunities for investing in human capital; and (4) discuss topics and priority areas for the National Academies. In the same year, the National Academy of Medicine (NAM) launched its Culture of Health Program to focus on the cultural factors that give rise to health inequities.

The NAM's Culture of Health Program is a multiyear collaborative effort, supported by the Robert Wood Johnson Foundation, to identify strategies to create and sustain conditions that support equitable good health for all Americans. On January 25, 2017, the NAM hosted its first stakeholder meeting of the program, "Engaging Allies in the Culture of Health Movement." The meeting brought together participants from major stakeholder groups, including philanthropy, membership associations, advocacy groups, community organizations, federal and state government, business leaders, and others not traditionally engaged with health equity issues. Presentations and discussions included health inequity across boundaries; early life inequities; and findings and recommendations from the first study of the program, *Communities in Action: Pathways to Health Equity.* The meeting concluded with a call to action to build a culture of health movement by empowering communities and working across sectors and disciplines.

An outcome of these two meetings is an edited volume of papers, *Perspectives on Health Equity and Social Determinants of Health*. This collection represents a variety of disciplines and varied schools of thought, and each paper includes a set of the authors' recommendations to advance the agenda to promote health equity for all.

The series is organized by research approaches and policy implications, systems that perpetuate or ameliorate health disparities, and specific examples of the ways disparities manifest in communities of color. Marks and colleagues lead off with an overview of the *Social and Structural Determinants of Health and Health Equity*, followed by a section on health equity research and policy. The section leads with a discussion of the relevance of *Health Inequities, Social Determinants, and Intersectionality* in promoting health equity and social justice (López and Gadsden). An underlying theme is underscored by Tolan et al. in holding that "health equity should be as central if not more so than any other concern, principle, criterion, or value in any national prioritizing of scientific agenda, health status and care goals, knowledge organization and evaluation, practice advisories, and/or policy formulations." They maintain that health equity is as essential a form of justice as equity in criminal and civil legal protections. Young follows this by drawing a connection between poverty and how *The Character Assassination of Black Males* can lead to detrimental consequences for public health research. This section continues by providing examples and guidance on how to promote health equity through research and policy, including by dismantling genetic determinism (Lerner). Seidel and colleagues emphasize the need to clearly delineate, conceptually and operationally, the meaning of equity, through an examination of ways inequities are perpetuated in *Philosophical Perspectives on Social Justice*.

Systems play a critical role in decreasing health disparities and increasing equity. The second section begins with a discussion by Meek and Gilliam on how school disciplinary strategies lead to later life problems, including health-compromising behaviors among children of color. Hutchinson and colleagues draw upon the important lessons we can learn from military medicine in *Lessons for Health Equity: Military Medicine as a Window to Universal Health Insurance*, and *Principles of Adolescent- and Young-Adult-Friendly Care* imparts equally important lessons that can be translated to medical settings serving marginalized youth (Diaz and Peake).

The series concludes with a section on the implications of health inequities in different populations and communities of color. Dill-Shackleford and colleagues emphasize the media's role in the portrayal of black men and how this can lead to harmful health consequences. Mokuau and colleagues give a powerful voice to an often-overlooked community in exploring the *Challenges and Promise of*

Health Equity for Native Hawaiians and Bell highlights the increased prevalence of fetal alcohol spectrum disorders in low-income African American communities. Finally, *Urgent Dispatch: Calling on Leadership to Respond to Violence in Black Neighborhoods* is a poignant examination of how we should engage leaders as central influential voices for change (Toomer and Mack).

The rich discussions found throughout make way for the translation of policies and actions to improve health and health equity for all citizens of our society. The major health problems of our time cannot be solved alone. Collective action is needed and it is needed now. It is the responsibility and duty of everyone to build a culture of health where all people have a chance at the healthiest life possible.

—Kimber Bogard, Velma McBride Murry,
and Charlee Alexander, *Editors*
March 2018

ACKNOWLEDGMENTS

We are humbled by the unwavering commitment of our authors and reviewers to raising visibility around barriers to achieving health equity, and promoting solutions for building a more equitable society. Thank you to all of you for your hard work and collaboration. We also thank Kaitlyn Friedman, Vanderbilt University, and Rajadhar Reddy, The University of Texas at Dallas, two former fellows of the Innovation to Incubation Program at the National Academy of Medicine, who helped shepherd this collection of perspectives to completion. A special thank you to the members and staff of the National Academies' Roundtable on the Promotion of Health Equity and the Elimination of Health Disparities for their guidance and leadership on this critical issue.

CONTENTS

INTRODUCTION:

SOCIAL AND STRUCTURAL DETERMINANTS OF HEALTH AND HEALTH EQUITY

James Marks, MD, MPH, Helene Gayle, MD, MPH, and Dwayne Proctor, PhD

The National Academy of Medicine's (NAM's) leadership is of central importance to progress on recognition, understanding, and engagement of the health impact of social factors, signals, and biases in shaping health inequities, including racism and embedded poverty—the structural determinants of health inequity. The committee members and staff who prepared the recently released report on community-based solutions to promote health equity, *Communities in Action: Pathways to Health Equity*, underscored the reality and the power of these factors.[1] That is a fundamental statement and it is important for the nation to be aware that it is a conclusion supported by the NAM, and it is a conclusion derived from the committee's careful review of the profile and science of inequity.

The committee has also contributed a hopeful element, one stemming from examples selected from around the country on what nine communities are doing to engage key factors in health and health equity. At the January 2017 meeting convened by the NAM, "Engaging Allies in the Culture of Health Movement," stakeholders from across several sectors, including community organizations, research, philanthropy, and government, came together to consider the findings of the report and to explore the ways collaborative action could reverse the debilitating and lethal consequences of inequity. The discussion was rich and offered many insights important to our work together.

Health disparities and inequities have been experienced between and among people and communities since the earliest times that people began to organize themselves into groups and communities. In fact, some of the major factors motivating people to form communities related to the need to buffer threats to

---

1 National Academies of Sciences, Engineering, and Medicine. 2017. *Communities in action: Pathways to health equity*. Washington, DC: The National Academies Press. doi: 10.17226/24624.

health and safety. The recognition of the existence of disparities has prompted the development of scientific disciplines to study them.

In public health, the iconic John Snow investigation in London in the mid-1800s is an important example. He mapped the deaths from cholera during an epidemic and he found that the people who lived near and got their water from the Broad Street pump were more likely to become ill and die than people who lived elsewhere. His map and investigation was, at its core, about noticing a disparity, a difference between neighborhoods in deaths from cholera, and then taking action by removing the pump handle from the Broad Street well pump. He did it with the permission of the St. James Parish Board. In effect, he had to go to the official agency and get a policy decision. So, the very core of public health is observing a disparity—in this case, not between racial and ethnic groups probably and likely not even between education levels, but a disparity nonetheless—and then taking action.

William Foege, former Director of the Centers for Disease Control and Prevention, former President of the American Public Health Association (APHA), and member of the NAM, said in his APHA Presidential Address, "The philosophy of public health is social justice, and the primary goal of public health is to reduce or eliminate differences in mortality and morbidity between populations" (Foege, 1987). In so many words, he stated that disparity reduction, regardless of its source, in striving for equity in health is not part of what our field is about. It is our field's central purpose and fundamental goal. We often focus on race and income and education because health and well-being differences are linked to them in large, persistent, pervasive, and systemic ways, affecting almost every disease and injury.

The importance of health equity—of fairness—to health is of such centrality that it motivated the Robert Wood Johnson Foundation, where two of us work, to place the challenge of culture of health at the top of our agenda. Our focus in this respect is essentially about fairness, especially fairness in the opportunities for good health—the affordability, the safety, and the convenience of healthy choices in all aspects of our lives. It is about equity in health itself insofar as possible, not between individuals but between groups of people where basic biological differences cannot be blamed for that disparity. This is true within our borders, and on the global scene as well, where one of us (Helene Gayle) served as the head of CARE for nearly decade, leading work to combat fundamental inequities.

As leaders in health, we have to speak to the responsibility our nation has to everyone, with a special responsibility for those at great risk or in great need. Martin Luther King Jr. said, "Injustice anywhere is a threat to justice everywhere." Translated to health, this means that when injustice is unchallenged, including the injustice of health disparities anywhere, society exposes its shared sense of community and nationhood to imminent risk of corrosion. These realities underscore the importance of the Academies' report and the subsequent meeting. The *Communities in Action* report clearly outlines that health inequities are in large part a result of poverty, structural racism, and discrimination, and that disparities based on race and ethnicity are the most persistent and difficult to address. In fact, the committee's Recommendation 3-1 calls for funders to support additional research on the multiple effects of structural racism and implicit and explicit bias on health and health care delivery. The report also recognizes that discrimination extends beyond race, and that many groups—women, the LGBTQ community, people who are poor, the undereducated, and those with mental and physical delays and disabilities—face discriminatory treatment and are subject to discriminatory policies. Solutions to improving health equity require additional research to understand how discrimination affects health.

Both the report and the conversation at the meeting recognize the relationship among health, equity, and hope. People with hope can and do make different decisions for themselves and their families than those that are without. And, hope can be studied, even like a vaccine. Mothers in Oklahoma, some of them with a new baby, were given a $1,000 college fund, a 529 plan, and others were not. Even though the cost of college is orders of magnitude beyond $1,000, it was found in this study that, by age 5, the children of mothers who had received the $1,000 529 plan were working better with others, were more kindergarten-ready, and the mothers themselves thought differently about their children's future (Beverly et al., 2016).

Even as we think of health equity as the outcome, we know that health and well-being are nurtured, they are protected and preserved, where people live, learn, work, and play. These are circumstances that our academic colleagues term the "social determinants of health," and it is in our communities that they play out. Throughout the discussions at the NAM meeting, time and time again, we heard reference made to the centrality and potential of community initiatives, whether the issue is getting children off on equal footing in life, better training and deploying human capital for progress, enlisting business to lead change, reinforcing communication strategies, and even drawing on design as a tool to improve health equity. A core assumption throughout each of the conversations was the need to recenter focus on communities, including the measures to guide and register progress.

Early childhood. Many participants emphasized beginning, even before birth, with efforts to produce equitable health prospects. Science yields daily insights about the importance of early environments to brain development, including lifelong implications for strengths, deficits, and resilience, underscoring the importance of prevention, and early intervention. James Comer's work to organize schools and communities around child development was called to mind, as were more recently reported results from birthing centers and early education centers, parental training, and support (https://medicine.yale.edu/childstudy/comer).

Human capital. With such influence increasingly ascribed to childhood experiences, emphasis on the capacity for stewardship on those experiences is vital. Support and training are needed for parents raising children in difficult circumstances, and, where parental challenges are incapacitating, alternative trusting relationships must be established. Descriptions were offered of a variety of strategies, including roles for grandparents, Head Start leaders, coaches, and guidance counselors. Examples given of supportive resources ranged from private grant programs such as that of the American Education Research Association to elements of the federal Potential in Every Student Succeeds Act to advance physical education, social, and mental health.

Communication. In our time of 24-7 connectedness, creative use of communications strategies offers a rapidly emerging and changing tool influencing culture and equity, hopefully a tool to be used with positive effect. It was noted that perhaps social media may be "the new barber shop or beauty parlor" as a means of helping to link and reach people with assistance. The example was given of the use of social media to encourage and assist young mothers in obtaining prenatal care.

Technology. As technology continues its rapid pace of development, opportunities are offered to equalize social and geographic access to resources that can potentially reduce disparities in access to diagnosis and treatment (e.g., rural communities) but can also facilitate broader dialogue within and among communities, and provide access to health-promoting applications from the gaming and app industries. The example was given of Go Noodle, a company aimed at promoting physical activity in schools, as was the case of using FaceTime capacity for grandparents to read to grandchildren from remote sites.

Design. Several references were made to the importance of the built environment—from the perspective of both perceptions and opportunities—in helping to reduce disparities. The American Planning Association and the American Institute of Architects are both organizations developing new commitments to elevating health concerns to a position of central consideration for their respective professionals. Programs such as the Safe Routes to Schools and Vision Zero community safety programs are good examples.

Business leadership. Economic vitality is the first order priority for any community and the businesses that shape its prospects. As a result, financial realism was also a feature of the meeting's conversations. Examples were given of prominent companies providing local-level leadership for progress, and especially encouraging were successful efforts to align health and business interests, noted in Just Causes' List of 100. Although the need of business to focus on return on investment has been raised as an obstacle to their taking leadership in the social improvement domain, the interesting experiences of ReadyNation's pay-for-success models of investing in good policies was encouraging.

Community leadership. To take advantage of the increasingly apparent opportunities, a strong commitment to move away from the typically vertical orientation of activities and focus across organizations and communities is necessary. This is the focus of findings from the National Academies' nine-community study, and it was also mentioned in the work of the Richmond Memorial Health Foundation to devote its entire programming effort to working with the mayor and community leaders to build a culture of health and address social determinants of health with multiple sectors throughout Greater Richmond. Also noted was the work on collective impact organizations in southern Oregon, joining law enforcement, K-12 education, and other social agencies targeting health equity.

Data. Often underappreciated, clear in this meeting's conversations was the importance of developing the community data infrastructure to identify problems, guide programs, and monitor results. Accordingly, also important is the commitment to invest in capacity that focuses on the most important issues in a fashion that is reliable and comparable across sites.

We are at a watershed time in our nation's history. We have to be honest with ourselves. Technologic advancement, where our nation's leadership is unquestioned, has not managed to rein in the growth in medical care costs, nor has it even enabled us to have better health relative to other countries of similar wealth and development according to standard, big-picture measures like life expectancy and infant mortality.

The major health problems of our time, especially as related to fairness and equity in health and well-being, cannot be solved by health care alone. They cannot be solved by public health alone. All of our nation's institutions—public, private, and nonprofit—have important roles to play even if they do not think of their purpose as being fundamentally about health and well-being. Every organization or sector of our society—business, health care, academia, schools, urban planning, parks and recreation, banking and finance, agriculture, childcare—has, as its core purpose, the value it brings to making a community a good place to live and to raise a family, so people can have warm relationships with neighbors and friends, enabling them to they can thrive and succeed.

As a nation, we have had an enormous imbalance regarding where we have looked for sources of health and illness and solutions to disparity. Some might have thought of the NAM as an unusual institution to ask to take a look at health and well-being for society as a whole, but the Academy can also speak to the heart about the values that are inherent in medicine and the protection of health.

Medicine has always been about the application of science to those who are in need, who are suffering, or who are at risk. There is an urgency to act even if the science is incomplete or immature. Each of us, from our own perspective, is grateful to the NAM for its commitment to showing what we, all of us, as leaders in and of our nation can do to make working together for a culture of health and well-being the duty and privilege it is.

REFERENCES

Beverly, S. G., M. M. Clancy, and M. Sherraden. 2016. *Universal accounts at birth: Results from SEED for Oklahoma Kids*. Center for Social Development. https://csd.wustl.edu/Publications/Documents/RS16-07.pdf.

Foege, W. H. 1987. Public health: Moving from debt to legacy. *American Journal of Public Health* 77(10):1276-1278.

SECTION I: HEALTH EQUITY RESEARCH AND POLICY

1

HEALTH INEQUITIES, SOCIAL DETERMINANTS, AND INTERSECTIONALITY

Nancy López, PhD, and Vivian L. Gadsden, EdD

ABSTRACT

In this essay, we focus on the potential and promise that intersectionality holds as a lens for studying the social determinants of health, reducing health disparities, and promoting health equity and social justice. Research that engages intersectionality as a guiding conceptual, methodological, and praxis-oriented framework is focused on power dynamics, specifically the relationships between oppression and privilege that are intrinsic to societal practices. Intersectional knowledge projects aimed at studying this interplay within and across systems challenge the status quo. Whether reframing existing conceptualizations of power, implementing empirical research studies, or working with community organizations and global social movements, intersectional inquiry and praxis are designed to excavate the ways a person's multiple identities and social positions are embedded within systems of inequality. Intersectionality also is attentive to the need to link individual, institutional, and structural levels of power in a given sociohistorical context for advancing health equity and social justice.

HEALTH DISPARITIES, INEQUITY, AND SOCIAL DETERMINANTS: A BRIEF CONTEXT

The urgency to promote health, reduce health disparities, and address the social determinants of health is highlighted in countless reports (Hankivsky and Christoffersen, 2008; World Health Organization, 2006, 2015). In short, problems in health disrupt the human developmental process. They undermine the quality of life and opportunities for children, youth, and families, particularly those exposed to vulnerable circumstances. Despite incremental change within and across health-serving agencies and increased health education and scrutiny of patient care, we continue to see significant disparities in the quality of health and life options that children in racial and ethnic minority, low-income homes and neighborhoods experience (Bloche, 2001). Research has uncovered several interconnections between health and environmental and social factors (Chapman and Berggren, 2005; Thorpe and Kelley-Moore, 2013) but has not always shifted paradigms sufficiently to either disentangle intersecting inequalities or tease apart the ways social factors and structural barriers at once interlock to prevent meaningful and sustainable change.

In this essay, we focus on the potential and promise that intersectionality holds as a lens for studying the social determinants of health, reducing health disparities, and promoting health equity and social justice. Collins and Bilge (2016) describe intersectionality as follows:

A way of understanding and analyzing complexity in the word, in people, and in human experiences. The events and conditions of social and political life and the self can seldom be understood as shaped by one factor. They are shaped by many factors in diverse and mutually influencing ways. When it comes to social inequality, people's lives and the organization of power in a given society are better understood as being shaped not by a single axis of social division, be it race or gender or class, but by many axes that work together and influence each other. Intersectionality as an analytic tool gives people better access to the complexity of the world and of themselves . . . People use intersectionality as an analytic tool to solve problems that they or others around them face. (p. 2)

We ask: How do we engage in inquiry and praxis (action and reflection) that departs from the understanding that intersecting systems of oppression, including race/structural racism, class/capitalism, ethnicity/ethnocentrism, color/colorism, sex and gender/patriarchy, and sexual orientation/heterosexism, nationality and citizenship/nativism, disability/ableism, and other systemic oppressions intersect and interact to produce major differences in embodied, lived race-gender that shape the social determinants of health? How can we as scholars, researchers, and practitioners concerned with child and family well-being take seriously the reality of how intersecting systems of power produce lived race-gender-class and other social locations of disadvantage and develop an intersectionality health equity lens for advancing health equity inquiry, knowledge projects, and praxis?

We argue that the potential power of intersectionality as a transformational paradigm lies in two domains relevant to understanding social determinants.

First, it is a critical knowledge project that questions the status quo and raises questions about the meaning and relationship between different social categories and intersecting systems of privilege and oppression (Bowleg, 2008; Collins, 2008, 2015; Collins and Bilge, 2016; Hancock, 2016; McCall, 2001; Yuval-Davis, 2011). It also pushes against the idea of "blaming the victim"—the simplicity of explaining health or educational outcomes by attributing problems to individuals' genetics or cultural and social behaviors alone. Second, by focusing on power relations at the individual, institutional, and global levels and the convergence of experiences in a given sociohistorical context and situational landscape, it serves as an anchor to advance equity and social justice aims for marginalized communities that have experienced and continue to experience structural inequalities (Collins, 2008, 2009, 2015; Crenshaw, 1993; Weber, 2010). In both instances, researchers and practitioners cross traditional academic, sectoral, and disciplinary boundaries to reconceptualize a problem and combine methods from different disciplines (e.g., in interdisciplinary research), or they apply conceptualizations and methods from one discipline to closely examine issues in another (e.g., in transdisciplinary research, epistemologies, and methodologies).

There is growing evidence and professional wisdom to suggest that health disparities do not exist in isolation, but are part of a reciprocal and complex web of problems associated with inequality and inequity in education, housing, and employment (LaVeist and Isaac, 2013; Schultz and Mullings, 2006; Weber, 2010; Williams and Mohammed, 2013). These disparities affect the unborn child through social-emotional challenges such as maternal stress and diagnosed and undiagnosed medical problems, including higher prevalence of gestational and preexisting diabetes in some pregnant populations. In other cases, they are observable at birth, particularly pronounced when prenatal care is unavailable, when the importance of care is not understood fully, and when young children are not exposed to the cognitive and social-emotional stimulation needed to thrive. These and other problems are manifested in parental stress, for example, in mother-headed and two-parent, low-income, and immigrant households alike. Parent and family adversity may reduce the number and quality of resources available and life experiences for children and families in the early years and throughout the life course. Such adversity is exacerbated by structural barriers that limit employment opportunities, increase housing instability, and contribute to homelessness, and that constrain efforts by families to effect positive change.

Over the past 20 years, two major shifts in discussions of health disparities and inequity have spurred interest and research. One shift is the growth in and opportunities presented by interdisciplinary and transdisciplinary research (e.g., work extending from sociology and psychology to economics, among other fields) and cross-domain practice (e.g., medicine, education, and social work) (see Gadsden et al., 2015b; LaVeist and Isaac, 2013). The reach of interests in these issues can be found not only in the social and medical sciences but also in contemporary ethical, moral, and political philosophy, such as Sen et al.'s (2009) linking of health equity and agency, and their commentaries on the implications for social justice. A second shift has been the heightened attention to health determinants, more frequently called social determinants of health, instead of a biomedical model that solely focuses on the individual-level make-up and behaviors of patients as the source of health disparity. The report of the Commission on the Social Determinants of Health (CSDH, 2008) points to the importance of being attentive to the overlapping effects and simultaneity of intersecting inequalities and their implications for social determinants:

> *The poor health of the poor, the social gradient in health within countries, and the marked health inequities between countries are caused by the unequal distribution of power, income, goods, and services, globally and nationally, the consequent unfairness in the immediate, visible circumstances of people's lives—their access to health care, schools, and education, their conditions of work and leisure, their homes, communities, towns, or cities—and their chances of leading a flourishing life. This unequal distribution of health-damaging experiences is not in any sense a "natural" phenomenon, but is the result of a toxic combination of poor social policies and programmes, unfair economic arrangements, and bad politics. Together, the structural determinants and conditions of daily life constitute the social determinants of health and are responsible for a major part of health inequities between and within countries. (p. 1)*

In emerging conceptualizations of these social determinants, racism and discrimination are overwhelmingly significant factors, but are not the only critical dimensions related to identity to be considered (Williams and Mohammed, 2013). They are tied inextricably to multiple identities and social locations that children, youth, and adults assume, and define a context for health (Bauer et al., 2016; Brown et al., 2016). One might argue that there is no issue more important than ensuring health. How a person understands this point and is able to act upon it is determined by more than her or his cognitive ability to engage the idea. It is influenced as well by a range of dynamic and situational identities and social positions that are biological, cultural, and epigenetic; by social determinants (i.e., where people are born, grow up, work, and age, and interact with their changing environments); and by a person's social experiences and encounters, rather than solely her or his self-agency across a variety of social settings. Even individuals with the strongest work ethic and sense of agency, when faced with daily problems associated with intersectionality across any combination of racial, class, gender, sexual orientation, language, or disability systemic oppressions and discrimination, may find fighting against these inequalities daunting.

Several researchers have advocated for a new way of combining the insights and perspectives used in intersectional knowledge projects in order to move away from decontextualized, biomedical frameworks that often fetishize "cultural competence" as the panacea for structural intersecting inequalities (Viruell-Fuentes et al., 2012). Instead of getting distracted by the alleged "deficits" or "individual behaviors" of marginalized communities, they call for what Chapman and Berggren (2005) refer to as a "radical contextualization of the social determinants of health perspectives." Sen and colleagues (2009) acknowledge this shift:

> In addition to the obvious benefit of deepening our insights into social inequalities and how they interact, the study of intersectionality . . . has the potential to provide critical guidance for policies and programmes. By giving precise insights into who is affected and how, in different settings, it provides a scalpel for policies rather than the current hatchet. It enables policies and programmes to identify whom to focus on, whom to protect, what exactly to promote and why. It also provides a simple way to monitor and evaluate the impact of policies and programmes on different subgroups from the most disadvantaged through the middle layers to those with particular advantages. (p. 412)

Our objective in the remainder of this essay is to provide a discussion of the possibilities for innovation in conceptualization, methodologies, and practices that can promote human development and health equity through an "intersectionality health equity lens." We employ Jones's (2016) definition of health equity. Jones defines health equity as "the [active] assurance of optimal conditions for all people." Jones explains that we can get there by "valuing everyone equally, rectifying historic inequities and distributing resources according to need." Jones invites us to think deeply and critically about equity as a never-ending process that requires constant and ongoing vigilance and not just an outcome that once accomplished can be forgotten. Building on Jones's (2016) and Collins and Bilge's (2016) ideas about equity and intersectionality we define an intersectionality health equity lens as ongoing critical knowledge projects, inquiry, and praxis that can include research, teaching, and practice approaches that are attentive to the ways systems of inequality interlock to create conditions for either health equity or health inequities (Collins, 2008, 2015; Collins and Bilge, 2016; Crenshaw, 1993).

We also embrace Collins and Bilge's (2016) core ideas of intersectionality, namely a focus on inequality, relationality and connectedness, power, social context, complexity, and social justice. They use the analogy of "domains of power" to paint a picture of the way that power is visible at the "interpersonal" or individual level in terms of who is advantaged or disadvantaged at the level of social interactions. For example, individuals may experience privilege or disadvantages when searching for a job, housing, interacting with law enforcement, or even when accessing a voting booth. Collins and Bilge (2016) assert

> *Using intersectionality as an analytic lens highlights the multiple nature of individual identities and how varying combinations of class, gender, race, sexuality, and citizenship categories differentially position every individual. (p. 8)*

Collins and Bilge (2016) also underscore that we must always be attentive to the "disciplinary" level as a domain of power that organizes and regulates the lives of people in ways that echo our distinct social positions with regard to systems of oppression. For example, rules about who will or will not be seen at a medical office because of the ability to pay a copay, who will or will not be admitted to a domestic violence shelter based on their English proficiency, and who has access to a gifted classroom, based on IQ test scores that are rooted in eugenicist origins, will inevitably impact the conditions for the advancement of health equity (see also Crenshaw, 1993; Zuberi, 2001).

Collins and Bilge also invite us to reflect on how power is visible at the "cultural" level or in the realm of ideas, norms, and narratives. For Collins and Bilge (2016), ideas matter and how messages are manufactured creates explanations, justifications, or challenges to the status quo vis-à-vis inequalities. For instance, if the idea that racialized health inequalities are simply a matter of individual behavior, food ways, and choice, and that we live in a meritocracy, where your station in life is simply a matter of individual effort, then we are subscribing to what Bonilla-Silva refers to as "colorblind" racism or the belief that present-day realities of race gaps in health only mirror individual deficits of individuals or defective cultures.

The last arena where Collins and Bilge interrogate the dynamic of power includes the "structural" level or at the level of institutional arrangements, which interrogates how intersecting systems of institutionalized power, whether in the economy and labor market in terms of whose labor is valued and who is exploited, or at the political level in who is granted substantive citizenship rights and privileges and who is not, as well as at the level of who has access to structures of political power and influence, shapes the institutionalization of the conditions for health equity. For example, the struggle for sovereignty of indigenous people, as evidenced in the Standing Rock movement to protect indigenous land and water for generations in South Dakota provides a snapshot of the structural location of indigenous nations and capitalist neoliberal actors that are in a struggle to define the environmental context for current and future generations, which will have grave consequences for health justice for marginalized indigenous communities.

While an intersectionality health equity lens may inform or drive interdisciplinary or transdisciplinary research, it must also be considered as part of both the process of conceptualizing the problem and the product of research on the problem. Throughout this essay, readers should consider the potential applications of an intersectionality health equity lens, how its use enhances (or disrupts) our understanding of salient and longstanding issues, what might be learned from its use that will inform and deepen research and practice with children and families who are among the marginalized in society, and what types of intersectionality-focused approaches might lead to health access and equity. In the next section, we focus on the contributions of an intersectionality health equity lens for research and for promoting health equity.

AN "INTERSECTIONALITY HEALTH EQUITY LENS" FOR SOCIAL JUSTICE

When developing or applying an intersectionality health equity lens, the researcher engages in deep self-reflection that contextualizes and recognizes the ways race, gender, class, sexual orientation, disability, and other axes of inequality constitute intersecting systems of oppression. Such systems produce very different lived experiences for entire categories of people who are embedded within complex webs and social networks at different levels (e.g., family, neighborhood, and community as well as institutional and structural). These lived experiences can either enhance or challenge the developmental pathways of children through adulthood and the ability of parents and families to ensure a positive trajectory for their children. They affect both the individual child and the networks and communities in which children live and grow and that define their access to resources.

An intersectionality health equity lens for the purposes of our discussion takes on the broader, philosophical meaning attached to praxis as a process involving health, educational, and social service researchers and practitioners in not only self-reflection but also action. Critical self-reflection allows researchers and practitioners to continually and closely examine their own race, gender, class, sexual orientation, disability, language, nativity/citizenship and social position, and their relationship to systems of inequality as part of intersecting systems of oppression and privilege. It argues for researchers and practitioners to draw upon their own experiences with health inequities and discrimination, and to understand and respond to new or subtle forms of inequities and discrimination. These subtle forms of inequity and discrimination are sometimes so deeply embedded in and accepted as societal practices that they may be difficult to uncover, yet render many children and families hopeless. The interplay between and among relevant systems and the statuses accompanying power attributed to different ethnic, racial, cultural, and socioeconomic groups affect both individuals and their social networks (e.g., family, neighborhood, and community). They are tied directly to and within institutional and structural hierarchies.

Crenshaw (1993) points to the entrenched nature of inequity, underscoring the need for a useful paradigm in which to locate the issues faced by African American women and other racially stigmatized, visible minority women of color. Credited with creating a systematic analysis of the concept of intersectionality, Crenshaw (1993) urged readers to "map the margins" by focusing on those social locations that remain invisible. She argues that such invisibility results from a reliance on a mythical, universal "black experience" (e.g., when we assume that the default category is the "black male experience" and by the same token when we speak about "'women's experiences" and assume that all women's experiences are represented in white women's experience). In each of these dominant conceptualizations of the black [male] and [white] woman's experience, heteronormativity is the invisible structure.

Crenshaw (1993) also illustrates how language, and potentially nativity and citizenship status, can serve as other axes of stratification that have received less attention than race and class. To illustrate her point, Crenshaw flexes her intersectional lens to bring into sharp relief the effects of "good intentions" on the real lives of women. She demonstrates that, despite their good intentions, some domestic violence shelters may operate in ways that ignore the plight of immigrant women with children who may not speak English and are unable to access domestic violence shelters. It goes without saying that this would structurally exclude immigrant (both documented and undocumented) women and their children who do not speak English. "Nativism, English Only" categories are the invisible, yet real, structural barriers to addressing domestic violence in the aforementioned situation. By the same token, members of lesbian, gay, bisexual, transgender, queer, and in-transition (LGBTQI) communities may not face explicit rules about being barred from these services because of their gender identity, but if counselors and other providers assume that their clients are in heterosexual, gender-conforming relationships, heteronormativity can operate as another type of an informal barrier.

One might well ask, given the complex relationships in addressing identity, whether it is possible to create intersectionality-grounded projects that integrate the issues of race, class, gender, disability, and other identities, statuses, and social locations in research on health and well-being for the range of issues facing marginalized children, youth, and families. Although we do not have a simple response, we highlight the need to address the real or perceived complexity of creating such projects and allowing time and resources for them to be developed well and to be refined (Cacari-Stone et al., 2017; López et al., 2017a, 2018; Van Hattum et al., 2017). We similarly understand the limitations of relying on one-dimensional categories that are, at best, additive, for example, first race, then maybe class, then maybe gender, depending on the focus of the research. As the World Health Organization (2015) and several health researchers before (e.g., LaVeist and Isaac, 2013; Williams and Mohammed, 2013) suggest, understanding the social determinants of health requires a broad reach to identify, and respond to, the embedded and entrenched inequities of policies that are situated in place and context.

Intersectionality health equity lenses help us understand that every person's experience is fundamentally different than the experience of others, based on their unique identity and structural positions within systems of inequality and structural impediments (Feagin and Sikes, 1994; López, 2003, Nakano Glenn, 2002, 2015; Weber, 2010). More than just a theory or framework to be used selectively, it is a commitment to developing a relentlessly critical and self-reflective lens that begins with the premise that race, class, gender, and other axes of social identities are intertwined and mutually constitutive, and that such a lens can help advance health disparities research, practice, and leadership by making the invisible visible (López et al., 2017b; López, 2018).

INTEGRATING RACE, GENDER, CLASS, AND SEXUALITY AS LIVED EXPERIENCES: A CASE EXAMPLE

In considering intersectionality projects, we must be aware of the overwhelming inequities associated with longstanding problems of race and gender and the added problems of poverty and class—problems that have narrowed in some cases over time but where inequality persists. It should come as no surprise that an intersectionality-focused project might appear opaque or obscure initially, despite its potential to uncover the breadth of issues faced in ensuring health and well-being.

Imagine the year 2050, and all institutional data are derived from the critical insight offered by Bowleg (2008):

It is the analysis and interpretation of research findings within the sociohistorical context of structural inequality for groups positioned in social hierarchies of unequal power . . . . that best defines intersectionality research. (p. 323)

López (2013) proposes the "racialized-gendered social determinant of health" as a heuristic device or framework for centering the lives of marginalized communities. This framework consists of two major concepts: (1) "lived race-gender" and (2) "racialized-gendered pathways of embodiment." López (2003) offers an example of the enactment of these concepts in the minds and experiences of both the observer and the observed. For example, she makes explicit the ways race-gender disparities are enacted and experienced in school and society by young Dominican and Caribbean men and women in what she calls "New York Immigration and Racialization." Consider Orfelia's narrative on the public's perceptions of blacks, Hispanics, and whites and the differential result of their identities on these perceptions:

If you put on the news, anyone who does anything bad, if he's not Black, he's Hispanic . . . . You watch the news and you see that when any white guy does something, you won't see their face. They might just say it, and that's all. But if it's a Dominican, a Hispanic, a Black, they put him on for about two minutes, so that you can know him. (p. 23)

Orfelia points to the ways she has internalized race and gender stigma as dominant identity markers and their intersections with place (Queens in New York) and other intersectional identities such as immigrant and Spanish speaker. The mental health costs of feeling racially stigmatized may become embodied by many youth who also feel what sociologist W. E. B. DuBois coined in 1903 as the "double consciousness" experienced by blacks in the U.S. context or the sense of always being seen with contempt, pity, or disdain because of one's stigmatized status (DuBois, 1999; Vidal-Ortiz, 2005).[1]

López also underscores the dominance of race and gender identities, along with other identities (e.g., social class, sexual orientation, age, ethnicity and nativity, and legal status) that form the basis for education and health frameworks. She draws upon a personal example to demonstrate connections among race, gender, sexuality, and social class and the significance attached to heteronormativity (Box 1-1).

---

1   See also Gravlee (2009) on when race becomes embodied.

BOX 1–1
Contextualizing Lived Race-Gender and the Racialized-Gendered Social Determinants of Health

As the U.S.-born daughter of Spanish-speaking immigrants from the Dominican Republic, I grew up as the eldest of five children in public housing in the Lower East Side of Manhattan in New York City during the 1970s and 1980s. I also graduated from a de facto segregated public high school, one of the last large vocational schools for girls in New York City. My cousin, labeled a boy, was born in the Dominican Republic but came to New York at the age of five; they[2] also grew up in New York City public housing in the 1970s and 1980s. Yet, we faced quite different life-course contexts that shaped our health status and health outcomes. While we are both Afro Latinos and would be described as racially black, my cousin was darker-skinned than me, and thus colorism operated to shape their experiences in ways that highlight the effects of colorism even within communities that would be racialized as black (Gómez, 2000; Hunter, 2007; Monk, 2015). My cousin often confided in me, sharing many of the experiences they had with police harassment connected to the criminalization of many black and Latin@ neighborhoods, and race-gender profiling policies and practices that created real fear among boys of color and particularly those who are visibly racialized as black or brown. Later, as a visibly transgender AfroLatinx (e.g., dark-skinned, black Dominican, gender-nonconforming adult), my cousin faced the additional challenge of being gender-nonconforming. For example, at their twenty-first birthday, while dancing with their Latinx partner, my cousin donned silver-sequined sportswear with a matching baseball cap. I often wondered about how my cousin's racialized-gendered-gender-nonconforming and sexual identity and social positions shaped their lived experiences while walking down the street, while attending school, while seeking an apartment, while seeking employment, or even when seeking health care, and, of course, while interacting with law enforcement. The constellation of social determinants of health that my cousin faced was starkly different than my own and could account for the fact that while I am in my late 40s, married, and the mother of two children, my cousin passed in New York City due to a chronic liver disease before reaching the age of 45 (Cuevas et al., forthcoming; Johnson et al., 2017; Ortiz et al., 2015).

---

2 "They" or "their" is used to denote the gender history of the transgender person.

While race, gender, and class were overriding identities in the short narrative in Box 1-1, heteronormativity was the silent but overpowering lens for López and her cousin.[3] As López notes, the nature and type of her cousin's experiences in and out of school, within family and community contexts, and with stressors that were unnamed distinguished the two cousins. As she suggests through this anecdote, sexuality played only a small though apparently significant part in the everyday encounters that her cousin faced. What remains unanswered are questions about the ways race and gender (male and Dominican) played in her cousin's schooling, and the ways that gender nonconformance (what we now refer to as transgender identity) produced barriers to health access, care, prevention, and maintenance; to employment; to housing; and to the daily acceptances that allow individuals to maintain not just a healthy personal racial, gendered, class, ethnic, or sexual identity but also an identity that can be embraced in full in all social domains and situations that López's cousin traversed throughout their short life.

Focusing on López's cousin's experiences from a health equity perspective, several additional questions are raised: Did the health system fail her cousin, or was it the larger social system that did not accept their intersectional identities? To what degree do our current systems of data collection make her cousin's intersecting lived oppressions vis-à-vis race, national origin, class, sexuality, gender identity, and nativity invisible? If we collect data only on gender identity and not class, nativity, citizenship, ethnicity, language, and/or national origin, do we make some social locations invisible? Do we ignore the temporal element of identities across the life course? How would López's cousin's life experiences have been different if her cousin had been from an LGBTQI middle class, Dominican immigrant family that was light skinned, white-looking Latinx and not a visible minority? All of these data challenges are opportunities for establishing communities of practice committed to intersectionality praxis (action and reflection).[4] Bowleg (2008) provides us with critical epistemological, ontological, and methodological insights on advancing intersectional inquiry and praxis:

---

3   For more information on providing equitable health care services for diverse LGBTQI communities, see Vidal-Ortiz (2005), NBER (2012), and Johnson et al. (2017). For information on the difference between ethical accuracy for civil rights and aesthetic accuracy for compliance only and the value added for having a separate question on Hispanic origin and race for the 2020 Consensus, please see Johnson et al. (2017).

4   For more on the AfroLatin@ experience in the United States, see Román and Flores (2010); for more information on providing equitable health care services for diverse LGBTQI communities, see Ortiz et al. (2015); for more on segregation, see Vidal-Ortiz (2004), NBER (2012), and Saenz and Morales (2015).

I argue that a key dilemma for intersectionality researchers is that the additive (e.g., Black + Lesbian + Woman) versus intersectional (e.g., Black Lesbian Woman) assumption inherent in measurement and qualitative and quantitative data analyses contradicts the central tenet of intersectionality: social identities and inequality are interdependent for groups such as Black lesbians, not mutually exclusive. In light of this, interpretation becomes one of the most substantial tools in the intersectionality researcher's methodological toolbox. (p. 312)

In studying these and other questions related to health access and equity, drawing upon broad conceptualizations and nuanced analyses is important as is drawing upon conceptually complementary methodological approaches. The efficacy of rigorous quasi-experimental studies and of large, integrated datasets, including administrative data, in identifying and addressing multiple problems facing differing communities is clear. For example, Brown and colleagues (2016) examine the influence of the intersecting consequences of race-ethnicity, gender, socioeconomics status (SES), and age on health inequality with almost 13,000 (n = 12,976) whites, blacks, and Mexican Americans, based on panel data from the Health and Retirement Study. Drawing upon multiple-hierarchy stratification and life-course perspectives, they focus on (1) the variation of racial/ethnic stratification of health by gender and/or SES and (2) the decrease, stability, or increase of combined inequality in health between middle and late life. Analyses of the data indicated that the effects of racial/ethnic, gender, and SES stratification were interactive, resulting in the greatest racial/ethnic inequalities in health among women and those with higher SES.

Although improving our quantitative data infrastructure is of paramount importance, Chapman and Berggren (2005) also call upon health disparities researchers to take advantage of the benefits of qualitative data methods that "radically contextualize" the sociohistoric contexts that fuel the social determinants of health. They argue that qualitative methodologies such as participant observation, ethnography, and interviews can serve to demystify the link between structural, institutional, community, and individual processes that contribute to health inequities by shedding light on the social practices, interactions, policies, mechanisms, and processes that undergird manufactured health inequities. Rather than committing to one or the other, this focus on intersectionality will require the use of multiple methods, strategically layered to identify the problem and provide responsive interventions and equitable policies (Minkler and Wallerstein, 2011).

An intersectional paradigm or conceptual universe takes identity categories embedded within systems of inequality as a starting point to understanding the interactions between individuals and systems and among individual identities, systems, and social locations across the life course. The categories are fluid and must be examined in combination with each other. Metzl and Hansen's (2014) concept of "structural competency" offers a useful example. It begins with the assumption that "inequalities in health [education, employment, housing, voting, law enforcement, nativity, etc.] must be conceptualized in relation to the institutions and social conditions that determine . . . resources" (p. 127). Discussions of intersectionality address Metzl and Hansen's concerns, described earlier, and emphasize the importance of examining the simultaneity of racism, sexism, heterosexism, classicism, and other axes of inequality for mapping and interrupting the sedimentation of health inequities in health care access and the social determinants of health. This perspective is moving slowly into mainstream health disparities research, as health focuses more directly on the social bases for health determinants (WHO, 2015). Intersectionality considers the multiplicity of policies and practices constructed for different groups. At the same time, it acknowledges the ways these historically situated policies and practices reinscribe positions of power, dominance, and oppression that contribute to the social determinants of health, education, and well-being.

DEVELOPING AN INTERSECTIONALITY HEALTH EQUITY LENS: CHANGING THE NARRATIVE FOR SOCIAL JUSTICE

What happens when health research takes an intersectional stance in producing and using knowledge to effect positive practice and social change and advance equity? In what ways do our personal and professional positionalities contribute to this intersectional stance, our research, and the opportunities afforded by our ways of seeing and knowing the world? How do we address the health inequalities and inequities that reduce these opportunities for children, youth, and families and redirect them to promote social justice?

We are aware that the answers to these questions require time, depth of inquiry, and breadth of analysis, and that they contribute to, rather than outline, a social justice framework. Throughout this essay, we argue that a critical, self-reflexive intersectionality health equity lens and praxis depend upon a visceral commitment to uncovering the workings of the multiple systems of inequality in unpacking the social determinants of health. Such a lens might be expanded to become an "intersectionality equity" lens that questions further how our research, teaching, and practice can enact Crenshaw's (1993) idea of "mapping the margins." To achieve this, Crenshaw argues, we must center the lives of groups that remain often invisible when we talk about the generic working class "women" or "men" or "Latinos" or "LGBTQ" communities.

In moving forward, we also must be committed to enlarging and diversifying the pool of research scientists who study the issues. By diversity within an intersectionality health equity lens, we are referring to research scientists whose own awareness of their intersectional identities—that is, ethnicity, race, gender, class, sexuality, nativity, and disability—pushes them to design research that produces greater knowledge and clarity about the conceptualization of sound intersectionality-grounded studies and the range of methods to ensure new knowledge, better applications of knowledge, and effective uses of knowledge to guide our understanding of human development and health.

Initiatives focused on advancing social cohesion through intentional efforts to increase the diversity and number of research scientists with lived experiences that reflect multiple intersecting systems of oppression may take different forms. For example, in April 2011, the Institute for the Study of "Race" and Social Justice at the University of New Mexico, with support from a National Institutes of Health workshop grant, convened a group of scholars from the health and biological sciences and social sciences who embodied the intersecting race, gender, sexual orientation, class, age, disability status, religious, ethnic, citizenship, and national origin backgrounds that form the rich tapestry of our diverse union (Figure 1-1).

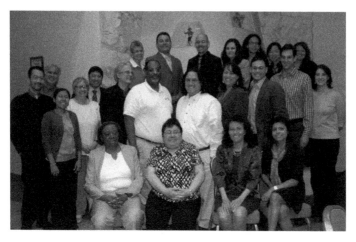

FIGURE 1-1 | National Institutes of Health (NIH) R21 Workshop. This gathering convened diverse multidisciplinary scholars for a workshop entitled, "Mapping 'Race' & Inequality: Best Practices for Conceptualizing and Operationalizing 'Race' in Health Policy Research Workshop," April 29–30, 2011. The Institute for the Study of "Race" and Social Justice, RWJF Center For Health Policy, University of New Mexico, Albuquerque, NM, convened the workshop. Papers from this workshop were published in Gómez and López (2013).

Other activities may include opportunities for interdisciplinary conferences and collaborative research, teaching, and writing. For example, at the University of Pennsylvania, one health disparities course is cofacilitated with tenure-track and clinical faculty within education and across the social sciences, medicine, and nursing. Bringing together all of the insights from health sciences, psychology, anthropology, art history, American studies, and law can actually generate new knowledge and new ways of doing research and developing equity-based policy. It is tremendously powerful to build on interdisciplinary knowledge. It is not the case that any one discipline has all the answers. We need all of us working together, harmoniously, to continue to make advancements and these insights should be reflected in what is considered required coursework for all disciplines interested in health equity.

An intersectionality health equity lens offers enormous possibilities for research projects that take seriously the multiple identities of children, youth, and families in the study of health and human development. One might argue that a relationship exists between social-ecological models of human development and health that highlight the intersections and interactions between and across contexts and discussions of intersectionality that consider social statuses.

In supporting an "intersectionality health equity lens" for research, we accept the limitations of implementation and of ways of looking at problems that children, youth, and families face. In our examples, drawn from our personal and research experiences, we suggest that there is little to no likelihood that a clean, one-size-fits-all approach exists to uncover the multiple intersectional identities in a given situation or sociopolitical and historical context. We also argue that to reveal the full expanse of complex intersecting factors that create social determinants of health and well-being, the discomforts associated with linking the different identities, the tendency to focus on one over another, and the difficulty of determining and building appropriate methodologies will have to be addressed (see Gadsden et al., 2014, 2015a). Palència and colleagues (2014), referring to their research and practice in Barcelona, remind us that "the development of research designs and methods that capture effectively all of the tenets of intersectionality theory remains underexplored" (p. 8). While intersectional analyses have relied heavily on ethnographic approaches, the authors note that "quantitative researchers have acknowledged the tensions between conventional research designs, intended to test for independent effects, and intersectionality principles" (p. 8).

The social sciences and health sciences are making progress toward considering the range of factors outside of simple genetics and social environments that affect health and health interventions. Intersectionality knowledge projects draw upon

BOX 1-2
Partial List of Intersectionality-Focused Resources

Columbia University
Center for Intersectionality and Social Policy Studies, established in 2011
Professor Kimberlè Crenshaw, Executive Director and Founder
http://www.law.columbia.edu/centers/intersectionality/about-the-center

University of Maryland
Consortium on Race, Gender and Ethnicity (CRGE), established in 2001
Dr. Ruth Zambrana, Director
http://crge.umd.edu

Matrix Center for the Advancement of Social Equity and Inclusion, established 2005
University of Colorado, Colorado Springs
Dr. Abby Ferber
http://www.uccs.edu/~matrix

University of New Mexico
New Mexico Race, Gender Class Data Policy Consortium, established 2014
Institute for the Study of "Race" and Social Justice, established 2009
Dr. Nancy López, Director and Cofounder
http://race.unm.edu

University of New Orleans
Race, Gender and Class Journal, established 1996
Dr. Jean Ait Belkhir, Director and Founder
http://rgc.uno.edu/journal

University of Southern California
Research Institute for the Study of Intersectionality and Social Transformation, established 2016
Dr. Ange Marie Hancock, Executive Director and Founder
http://www.ange-mariehancock.com

Simon Fraser University
Institute for Intersectionality Research and Policy, established 2005
Dr. Olena Hankivsky, Director
http://www.sfu.ca/iirp/

Anna Julia Cooper Center
Advancing Justice Through Intersectional Scholarship
Wake Forest University
Dr. Melissa Harris Perry, Director
http://ajccenter.wfu.edu

and have the potential to create innovative research and policy paradigms that can lead to practical measures and solutions for advancing health equity. Such measures map and interrupt inequality among racially stigmatized and other marginalized communities in local, municipal, state, and national contexts. At a minimum, they suggest a revisioning of policies that cut across relevant areas of health, education, social services, and law.

In developing our focus on intersectionality and social determinants of health, we attach our analysis to the goals of advancing social justice, where commitments to equality and equity reside and power is shared. A list of resources focused on intersectionality appears in Box 1-2 and demonstrates the range of efforts. As these efforts suggest, for all health and health policy researchers, scholars, practitioners, and community leaders who embrace a social justice framework, an intersectionality health equity lens could help to illuminate the often stifled issues that affect the health, development, and well-being of children and families in marginalized communities. This would mean that they would take seriously the ways institutional rights and duties allow people to participate and receive resources such as health, education, and social services in ways that are fundamentally shaped by intersecting inequalities. That would also mean promoting equal access to the fair distribution of wealth, equal opportunity, and equality of outcome by making the invisible visible through interrogating how race and class systems of oppression work together in shaping the social determinants of health.

Organizations such as the NAM can serve as convergence spaces where intersectionality knowledge projects centering on the lives of multiple and diverse marginalized groups in a given sociohistorical context can be incubated and developed to advance health justice. How specialists see, treat, and understand the human experiences of children and families and the potential for their well-being will be revised. As a result, we begin to address the multiplicity of identities, social positions, and systems of intersecting inequalities that contribute to the social determinants of health for diverse populations of children, youth, and families and move closer to effecting sustainable change and equity.

REFERENCES

Bauer, G. 2014. Incorporating intersectionality theory into population health research methodology: Challenges and the potential to advance health equity. *Social Science and Medicine* 110:10–17.

Bloche, M. G. 2001. Race and discretion in American medicine. *Yale Journal of Health Policy, Law, and Ethics* 1(1):5.

Bowleg, L. 2008. The methodological challenges of qualitative and quantitative inter-sectionality research. *Sex Roles* 59:312-325.

Brown, T. H., L. J. Richardson, T. W. Hargrove, and C. S. Thomas. 2016. Using multiple-hierarchy stratification and life course approaches to understand health inequalities: The intersecting consequences of race, gender, SES, and age. *Journal of Health and Social Behavior* 57(2):200-222.

Cacari-Stone, L., C. Diaz Fuentes, N. López, F. Raj Joshi, and M. Lauvidaus. 2017. The heart of gender justice in New Mexico: Intersectionality, economic security, and health equity (Part 2: Quantitative data analysis). Santa Fe, NM: NewMexicoWomen.org.

Chapman, R., and J. Berggren. 2005. Radical contextualization: Contributions to an anthropology of racial/ethnic health disparities. *Health: An Interdisciplinary Journal for the Social Study of Health, Illness, and Medicine* 9(2):145–167.

Collins, P. H. 2008. *Black feminist thought: Knowledge, consciousness, and the politics of empowerment.* New York: Routledge.

Collins, P. H. 2009. *Another kind of public education: Race, schools, the media and democratic possibilities.* Boston, MA: Beacon Press.

Collins, P. H. 2015. Intersectionality's definitional dilemmas. *Annual Review of Sociology* 41:1–20.

Collins, P. H., and S. Bilge. 2016. *Intersectionality.* Malden, MA: Polity Press.

Crenshaw, K. 1993. Mapping the margins: Intersectionality, identity politics, and violence against women of color. In *Critical race theory: The key writings that formed the movement,* edited by K. Crenshaw, N. Gotanda, G. Peller, and K. Thomas. New York: New Press. Pp. 357–383.

CSDH (Commission on Social Determinants of Health). 2007. *Building a global move-ment for health equity.* World Health Organization. Available at: http://www.who.int/social_determinants/resources/csdh_media/csdh_interim_statement_07.pdf.

CSDH. 2008. *Closing the gap in a generation: Health equity through action on the social deter-minants of health.* Final Report. Geneva: World Health Organization.

Cuevas, A., K. Ortiz, N. López, and D. Williams. Assessing racial differences in lifetime and current smoking status & menthol consumption among Latinos in a nationally representative sample. *Ethnicity and Health,* forthcoming.

DuBois, W. E. B. 1999. On spiritual strivings. In *The souls of black folk,* edited by H. L. Gates and T. H. Oliver. New York: W. W. Norton and Company.

Feagin, J. R., and M. P. Sikes. 1994. *Living with racism: The black middle-class experience.* Boston, MA: Beacon Press.

Gadsden, V., D. Gioia, and K. Mostafa. 2014. *Shifting the conversation: Emotional labor as learning in a pedagogy of discomfort.* Poster presented at the 2014 American Educational Research Association Annual Meeting, Philadelphia, PA.

Gadsden, V., K. B. Jacobs, and N. Peterman. 2015a. *Emotion, knowledge, and inquiry: Students' comforts and discomforts in studying race, culture, and equity.* Paper presented at the American Educational Research Association Annual Meeting, Chicago, IL.

Gadsden, V. L., N. Peterman, R. Maton, M. Yee, and M. Johnston. 2015b. *University-community health partnerships: An inquiry into family and community health beliefs and practices.* Paper pre-sented at the American Educational Research Association Annual Meeting. Chicago, IL.

Glenn, E. 2002. *Unequal freedom: How race and gender shaped American citizenship and labor.* Boston, MA: Harvard University Press.

Glenn, E. N. 2015. Settler colonialism as structure: A framework for comparative studies of US race and gender formation. *Sociology of Race and Ethnicity* 1(1):52-72.

Gómez, L. E. (2000). Race, colonialism, and criminal law: Mexicans and the American criminal justice system in territorial New Mexico. *Law and Society Review,* 1129–1202.

Gómez, L. E., and N. López, eds. 2013. *Mapping "race": Critical approaches to health disparities research.* New Brunswick, NJ: Rutgers University Press.

Gravlee, C. 2009. How race becomes biology: Embodiment of social inequality. *American Journal of Physical Anthropology* 139:47–57.

Hancock, A. M. 2016. *Intersectionality: An intellectual history.* Oxford University Press

Hankivsky, O., and A. Christoffersen. 2008. Intersectionality and the determinants of health: A Canadian perspective. *Critical Public Health* 18(3):271–283.

Hunter, M. 2007. The persistent problem of colorism: Skin tone, status, and inequality. *Sociology Compass* 1(1):237–254.

Johnson III, R. G., M. Rivera, and N. López. 2017. Social movements and the need for a trans ethics approach to LGBTQ homeless youth. *Public Integrity* 19:1-14.

Jones, C. 2016. Closing General Session, "Creating the Healthiest Nation: Ensuring the Right to Health." American Public Health Association Annual Meeting, Denver, CO.

LaVeist, T. A., and L. Isaac, eds. 2013. *Race, ethnicity, and health,* 2nd ed. San Francisco, CA: Jossey-Bass.

López, N. 2003. *Hopeful girls, troubled boys: Race and gender disparity in urban education.* New York: Routledge.

López, N. 2013. Contextualizing lived race-gender and the racialized gendered social determinants of health. In *Mapping "race": Critical approaches to health disparities research,* edited by L. Gómez and N. López. New Brunswick, NJ: Rutgers University Press. Pp. 179–211.

López, N. 2017b. Why the 2020 Census should keep longstanding separate questions about Hispanic origin and race. *Scholars Strategy Network.* Available from http://www.scholarsstrategynetwork.org/brief/why-2020-census-should-keep-longstanding-separate-questions-about-hispanic-origin-and-race.

López, N. 2018. The US Census Bureau keeps confusing race and ethnicity. *The Conversation,* February 28, https://theconversation.com/the-us-census-bureau-keeps-confusing-race-and-ethnicity-89649.

López, N., E. Vargas, M. Juarez, L. Cacari-Stone, and S. Bettez. 2017a. What's your "street race"? Leveraging multidimensional measures of race and intersectionality for examining physical and mental health status among Latinx. *Sociology of Race and Ethnicity,* doi:10.1177/2332649217708798.

López, N., C. Erwin, M. Binder, and M. Chavez. 2018a. Making the invisible visible through critical race theory and intersectionality: Race-gender-class gaps at a public university in the southwest 1980–2015. *Race, Ethnicity and Education,* 21:180-207.

McCall, L. 2001. *Complex inequality: Gender, class, and race in the new economy.* New York: Routledge.

Metzl, J., and H. Hansen. 2014. Structural competency: Theorizing a new medical engagement with stigma and inequality. *Social Science & Medicine* 103:126–133.

Minkler, M., and N. Wallerstein, Eds. 2011. *Community-based participatory research for health: From process to outcomes.* New York: John Wiley & Sons.

Morgen, A. 2006. Movement-grounded theory: Intersectional analysis of health inequalities in the U.S. In *Gender, race, class and health: Intersectional approaches,* edited by A. Schultz and L. Mullings. San Francisco, CA: Jossey-Bass. Pp. 394–423.

Monk, E. 2015. The cost of color: Skin color, discrimination, and health among African-Americans. *American Journal of Sociology* 121(2):1-49.

NBER (National Bureau of Economic Research). 2012. *A summary overview of Moving to Oppportunity: A random assignment housing mobility study in five U.S. cities.* Moving to Opportunity for Fair Housing Program, Department of Housing and Urban Development. Available from http://www.nber.org/mtopublic/MTO%20Overview%20Summary.pdf.

Ortiz, K. S., D. T. Duncan, J. R. Blosnich, R. G. Salloum, and J. Battle. 2015. Smoking among sexual minorities: Are there racial differences? *Nicotine & Tobacco Research* 17(11):1362–1368.

Palència, L., D. Malmusi, and C. Borrell. 2014. *Incorporating intersectionality in evaluation of policy impacts on health equity: A quick guide.* Agencia de Salut Publica de Barcelona. CIBERESP. Available from http://www.sophieproject.eu/pdf/Guide_intersectionality_SOPHIE.pdf.

Román, M. J., and J. Flores, eds. 2010. *The Afro-Latin@ reader: History and culture in the United States.* Durham, NC: Duke University Press.

Saenz, R., and M. C. Morales. 2015. *Latinos in the United States: Diversity and change.* John Wiley & Sons.

Schultz, A., and L. Mullings. 2006. Intersectionality and health: An introduction. In *Gender, race, class and health: Intersectional approaches,* edited by A. Schultz and L. Mullings. San Francisco, CA: Jossey-Bass. Pp. 3–20.

Sen, G., A. Iyer, and C. Mukherjee. 2009. A methodology to analyse the intersections of social inequalities in health. *Journal of Human Development and Capabilities* 10(3):397–415.

Thorpe, R., and J. Kelley-Moore. 2013. Life course theories of race disparities: A comparison of cumulative dis/advantage perspective and the weathering hypothesis. In *Race, ethnicity, and health,* edited by T. A. LaVeist and L. Isaac. San Francisco, CA: Jossey-Bass. Pp. 355–375.

Van Hattum, F., S. Ghiorse, and A. Villamil. 2017. *The heart of gender justice in New Mexico: Intersectionality, economic security, and health equity (Part 1: Community dialogues).* Santa Fe, NM: NewMexicoWomen.Org.

Vidal-Ortiz, S. 2004. On being a white person of color: Using autoethnography to understand Puerto Ricans' racialization. *Qualitative Sociology* 27(2):179–203.

Vidal-Ortiz, S. 2005. Sexuality and gender in Santería: LGBT identities at the crossroads of Santería religious practices and beliefs. In *Gay religion,* edited by S. Thumma and E. Gray. Walnut Creek, CA: Altamira Press. Pp. 115–138.

Viruell-Fuentes, E. A., P. Y. Miranda, and S. Abdulrahim. 2012. More than culture: Structural racism, intersectionality theory, and immigrant health. *Social Science & Medicine* 75(12):2099–2106.

Weber, L. 2010. Defining contested concepts. In *Understanding race, class, gender and sexuality: A conceptual framework*. New York: Oxford University Press. Pp. 23–43.

WHO (World Health Organization). 2006. *Constitution of the World Health Organization. Basic Documents*, 45th ed., Supplement. Available from http://www.who.int/governance/eb/who_constitution_en.pdf.

WHO. 2015. *Health systems equity update*. Available from http://www.who.int/healthsystems/topics/equity/en.

Williams, D., and S. Mohammed. 2013. Racism and health, I: Pathways & scientific evidence. *American Behavioral Scientist* 57(8):1152–1173.

Yuval-Davis, N. 2011. *The politics of belonging: Intersected contestations*. London, UK: Sage.

Zuberi, T. 2001. *Thicker than blood: How racial statistics lie*. Minneapolis, MN: University of Minnesota Press.

2

IDENTIFYING AND IMPLEMENTING OPPORTUNITIES TO REALIZE HEALTH EQUITY THROUGH A LIFE SPAN LENS OF LEGAL AND POLICY RESEARCH

Patrick H. Tolan, PhD, Velma McBride Murry, PhD, Angela Diaz, MD, PhD, MPH, and Robert Seidel, MLA

Our perspective is grounded in the proposition that health equity should be central or more significant than any other concern, principle, criterion, or value when prioritizing a national scientific agenda, setting care goals, organizing research and evaluation, and formulating practice advisories and policy. The lens of how a given topic or task relates to health equity or lack thereof should be front and center.

OVERARCHING FRAMEWORK

Use of this framework has the potential to advance health equity as a priority for our nation and entails not simply favoring diversity of samples, attending to epidemiological variations, and mounting good faith efforts for greater access to care for those with fewer resources, but encompasses the integration of health equity as fundamental in formulating specific scientific questions as well as framing the overall research agenda. Viewing health equity as a core concept of social justice includes tending to all aspects of scientific inquiry, including research designs and methods and the organizing, interpreting, and evaluating of scientific findings. We do not suggest that ideas presented here are novel, as we are not the first to argue for this approach (IOM, 2002; Moy et al., 2005; NRC, 2004; Sen, 2009). Nor do we claim to provide detailed comprehensive arguments addressing the numerous issues that arise in privileging this perspective over other frameworks that have emerged to address health equity and justice. With this disclaimer, we begin our discussion outlining the foundation, implications, and some key features of and basis for our position noted here, and will delve into a few of the primary ensuing implications.

DUAL TRACKS OF RESEARCH FOR CREATING HEALTH EQUITY

To advance our efforts to reduce health disparities through the elevation of health equity and justice, we suggest that two major tracks of scholarship serve as basic avenues of study: (1) application of highest-quality research from a life span developmental approach in studying causes, modifiers, trajectories, and outcomes related to health and disease and (2) empirical study and systematic policy analyses of regulations and laws and related procedures, criminal and civil, that affect health equity. This includes those that may in intention or practice impede health equity but also a vigorous search for identifying those that promote health equity. We contend that the parallel pursuit and connection between these two tracks would be advantageous so that health equity is central within biomedical and human development science and in the policy and laws affecting health opportunities and care. Additionally, this will help decrease the disparities based on ethnic group and economic class currently evident in health status, health opportunities, health services, and health outcomes.

These two tracks, research through a developmental lens and policy analysis, are rudimentary and limited instruments of knowledge development. Yet, despite their insufficiencies, they are appropriate tools for promoting the production of sound information to help mitigate this national crisis. In addition, this framework allows for the inclusion of multiple influences of health over the life span. Our thesis holds that in refining our understanding of how equity can be realized, or even how it is more aptly considered for guiding health policy, these twin pursuits of scholarship represent the most reliable pathways through the thickets of opinion, prejudice, disinterest, and haste that encumber alternative frameworks. Further, pursuit along these two lines of inquiry holds promise for the evolution of sound knowledge and true progress to health equity.

A second major proposition of this paper is to shift the formulation and evaluation of scientific work away from how research findings clarify disparities, toward an initial identification of how an issue or theory is formulated. This would advance knowledge about ways to facilitate health equity or minimize injustice and, in this instance, disparities. Clearly, having more detailed information about the actual mechanisms through which disparities in susceptibility to disease are linked to access to resources, treatment quality and availability, and life-course trajectories are critical for recognizing the extent of the inequity.

Such knowledge can inform and guide approaches and strategies to increase health equity and, in turn, promote justice.

Yet, beyond extensive documentation of these issues, there are numerous limitations to this approach. First, it can only imply need and potentially valuable actions in relation to current differences in inequity. Second, tracking and documenting history and risk patterns can inform but may provide little illumination about how risk patterns can be changed, prevented, shifted, and undone. We suggest, therefore, that at this juncture there is great advantage to giving preference to descriptive and experimental studies that illuminate how equity can be realized and the role of justice in this endeavor.

While perhaps appearing to reflect, simply, a grammatical "sleight of hand" or the other side of highlighting patterns and contributors to inequity, the impact of asking basic questions about how equity is or can be realized is the potential to bring new approaches to our understanding of health equity and justice—what is studied, how populations are identified and organized, how hypotheses are formulated, and what analyses are intended to reveal. The benefit of this approach is that what may seem a nuanced definitional refinement of health equity and justice can be profound, particularly in how the accumulated science is interpreted, and directs practice, policy, and next steps in scholarship.

DEFINING HEALTH EQUITY AND HEALTH DISPARITIES

The framework proposed and the emphases highlighted emanate from the juxtaposition of several conceptual elements that are prominent in the scientific and policy literature about health disparities and the aspiration of health equity (Braveman, 2006). Although one can find numerous definitions with different connotations of equity and how that relates to resource distribution (see Seidel et al., 2016), an operational definition has emerged that seems to specify what is meant by the term and what is not encompassed within that term. Health disparities refer to systematic health differences related to group membership (e.g., socioeconomic status, gender, and ethnic identity) and access to resources (knowledge, care, and practices) that are avoidable or malleable, and are primarily socially determined (Braveman, 2006; Whitehead, 1992). Thus, it is not just a matter of documenting health risk, status, use, or effect differences between groups or identifying individual instances of these but is reserved for *systematic differences* between groups that are related to social and associated political power and affect access to health opportunities, resources, and outcomes. A critical implication of this definition is that it proposes that systematic differences between groups can be affected or eliminated because they are representative of social and politically based inequities. Moreover, this perspective assumes, though not readily acknowledges, that these differences are essentially malleable. Further, an important corollary of this definition is that health equity is considered fundamental to social and civic justice and is based in the ethics of human rights (Daniels et al., 2009; Sen, 1999). This statement implies that because health equity is a fundamental right, all humans have the right to pursuit of life, and no one should have advantage over others by dint of position, historical legacy associated with ethnicity, gender, or social class in order to have access to health care services to be healthy and live out their natural life span (Bobinski, 2003). These perspectives are foundational in our pursuit of equity, justice, and human rights—values that our nation should uphold and actuate to eliminate disparities.

Health equity is as essential a form of justice as equity in criminal and civil legal protections. To raise the visibility of health equity as a matter of justice and ensure that all social groups have equal opportunity to reach their full potential to be as healthy as possible over their life span, there is need to reduce and eliminate systematic differences in the health of groups and communities whose poor health status is often due to social class and social positions in society (García Coll et al., 1996).

From this perspective, the standard or benchmark for health equity is the status enjoyed by those with substantial (above-average) privilege and/or access to resources, support, and care for health. This benchmark denotes what is plausible with adequate nurturance, care, support, and health promotion. As such, this benchmarking can be contrasted to a view that merely seeks to lessen gaps based on presumptions of differences in resource distribution or a view that seeks a lower level because it is presumed that increasing health status of those with lower status and economic capability will mean compromising health capabilities of those with greater privilege (Braveman, 2006; Seidel et al., 2016). Apart from or controlling for personal disposition, choices and practices, and familial-biological contributions, all persons, regardless of color, social class, social position, or physical/mental abilities, should enjoy the same quality of life, mortality probability, and opportunities for care, support, prevention, and promotive health care as others in our society (Marmot et al., 2008). For example, in its 2004 report, *Eliminating Health Disparities: Measurement and Needs*, the National Research Council noted that the infant mortality rate for African Americans was over twice that for European Americans (14.4/1,000 versus 5.7/1,000) but this difference could not be explained by differences in medical or nonsocial risk factors. To reduce this disparity, we suggest that identifying and instituting actions and policies that would reduce the infant mortality rate for African Americans so that they are similar to patterns occurring for European Americans should be the goal and focus for health equity in this area.

Braveman (2006, 2014) notes that the consideration of health equity grounded in fundamental human rights and establishing the benchmarks of those with considerable resources direct efforts toward identifying needs of those with lesser status and meeting those needs as a primary strategy for health equity. This approach is distinguished from a strategy of simply spreading access to resources as organized for and about those with privileged status. This approach should shift research, practice, funding, legal, and policy efforts away from merely ensuring that essentials are not inaccessible to identifying needs to attain equity, addressing systematic inequities for resource allocation, and benchmarking progress toward status for all, instead of continuing to reserve those resources for the most socially privileged.

A LIFESPAN DEVELOPMENT FRAMEWORK FOR HEALTH RESEARCH

Much of the health equity research to date has focused on documenting patterns of differences between groups in outcomes, exposure to risk factors, or differences in social and economic conditions that are thought to correspond to differences in health opportunities and resources. Although much of this work is consistent with a life-course perspective, the relation often has been implied or incidental. Our perspective is that a framework should be infused into the research agenda that identifies factors and processes that contribute to health promotion, with specific consideration given to identifying pathways to disease occurrence and preventive interventions—ones that offer health delivery services on a continuum ranging from promotion to prevention to treatment to maintenance. Further information advancing our understanding of variability in access to health-supporting care and resources is also needed. Similarly, this perspective can be informative in understanding how injustice and inequities in areas such as criminal justice, education, housing, employment, and political standing can influence health of groups. This would allow for a holistic, lifespan approach in our efforts to eradicate contributors to health inequities, thereby improving conditions that may hinder efforts to reduce and eventually eliminate health inequities (Braveman and Barclay, 2009).

The life-course perspective, as articulated here, focuses on longitudinal tracking over age and the connection of health contributors for a given person across time, and provides a systematic basis for understanding and explaining how prior life experiences and human development influence subsequent potentialities. The overarching assumption is that, to a great extent, early experiences have more profound shaping influence than later experiences, although not fully determining of later life course (Halfon and Hochstein, 2002; Lerner, 2006). Thus, one's health status is not only influenced by prior experiences from conception onward (and preconception genetic contributions, as well) but also is influenced by and manifested within a developmental ecology of social, environmental, and economic systems (Shanahan and Boardman, 2009). In turn, these affect one's social position regarding access to resources, exposure to impediments, and differential potentialities for healthier pathways that profoundly affect health equity (Bronfenbrenner and Morris, 2006).

The life-course framework maps out and describes the processes through which social structures impact individual lives, including biomedical, interpersonal, community, economic, legal, and political systems. It maps, describes, and explains the synchronic and diachronic distribution of individuals into social positions across their lifetime. This approach permits systematic, scientific, epidemiological studies that examine the linkages among microbiological aspects of health over time, within determinable typical or healthy processes to person-level behaviors and indicators that vary by demographic and economic groups. Further, this framework allows for the integration of social factors to explain disparities in opportunities for health; health-promoting influences; risk exposure and susceptibility; health orientation; health care access, quality, use, and attitudes; and likely pathways and outcomes of health practices, problems, and diseases. Using a comprehensive orientation to explain health also provides informative understanding of the links between accumulated risk across generations and systematic inequities due to a shared characteristic, such as how shared gender, ethnicity, or social class relates to advantage or disadvantage. Braveman (2014), for example, provides a detailed contrast between the lives of a young, impoverished, African American mother and a middle-income European American mother to illustrate a cascade of interdependent differences in opportunities, risks, control over health resources, and life circumstances that, in confluence, lead to quite divergent health status outcomes for the two women and their children. Braveman notes the difference in opportunity for prenatal care, advice and support for best neonatal parenting, likelihood of exposure to toxic chemicals during early childhood, safety of the neighborhood, economic stress during parenting years, quality of schools, and a cascade of differing environmental circumstances that culminate in substantial differences in morbidity and perhaps in lifespan. As one informative illustration, Braveman (2014) shows that, irrespective of particular interest, topic, or focus, a life-course perspective locates health research and actions within the transacting interdependent influences across biological, psychological, social, and societal systems. By doing so, oversimplifying the prioritization of one level of explanation over another is avoided, while multiple opportunities to affect inequities are identified. This approach keeps the malleability of health equity front and center.

A distinct advantage of the life-course perspective in explaining the systematic variations in individual and group health trajectories is that it provides opportunity to identify exceptions to overall patterns of inequity. It also allows for greater understanding of where equity is being realized or promoted, such as how, when, and where programs, practices, and policies are overcoming discriminatory practices, differential risk exposure, and constrained opportunity, and where opportunities exist to overcome or undercut inequity-promoting influences (Aaron and Chesley, 2003; Williams et al., 2013). For example, efforts to increase attention to implicit, cultural, and institutional racism in training of health providers have been shown to reduce inequities, in particular in the manner people of color are listened to and treated in health care service delivery systems (APHA, 2015). Similarly, by tracking the impact of access to better housing and neighborhoods with better educational and health resources, Acevedo-Garcia et al. (2004) found improved health status of persons of color from low-income communities, including lower rates of severe obesity and diabetes risk and higher rates of good mental health 10–15 years later (Ludwig et al., 2011, 2012). Another example is the Nurse Home Visiting Program, which provides young, low-income, mostly minority mothers with visits during pregnancy and the early childhood period. This program has demonstrated reductions in smoking during pregnancy, a known cause of low birth rate, behavioral problems, and multiple other health risks. In addition, rates of child abuse and neglect were reduced and the mothers were more likely to engage in employment programs and had lower arrest rates (Olds et al., 1997). The program had long-term indirect effects on the children over time, with lower arrest rates when they became adolescents. Thus, this program reduced health disparities in outcomes for these low-income mothers and their children. Another exemplar study was conducted by Tolan and colleagues (2016), who tested a program for inner-city families that promoted neighbor-to-neighbor connection of parents at the time their children entered first grade and supported parental school engagement as well as sharing of competencies in managing challenges of raising children in high-risk neighborhoods. The randomized controlled trial led to parents in the groups remaining involved in school while counterparts in the same schools and communities became less involved. According to follow-up conducted 11 years later, the program benefits translated to lower violence and behavioral problems for their children at school, with related lower substance use and risky sexual practices.

In addition, Murry and colleagues (2005) conducted a randomized trial of a universal preventive intervention to deter adolescent, risky sexual behavior, the Strong African American Families (SAAF) program, designed within the unique context of rural African American communities (Murry et al., 2005, 2014). The SAAF randomized controlled trial (667 families with an 11-year-old child) has successfully delayed both sexual debut and substance use, 54 months post-intervention (Brody et al., 2008; Murry et al., 2010), with sustaining HIV risk-reduction patterns of increased condom use and fewer sexual partners among sexually active SAAF youth, 65 months post-intervention (Murry et al., 2011, 2012). In addition, SAAF has demonstrated ripple effects on nontargeted areas, in particular, reduced depressive symptoms among parents, through the program's enhancement of positive parenting behaviors (e.g., consistent discipline, youth monitoring, and open communication) which, in turn, evinced improvement in child behavior (e.g., reduced conduct problems, parent–child arguing, and deviant peer affiliation; Beach et al., 2008). These results support the link between reduced depressive symptoms and stronger family relationships, particularly the importance of enhanced parenting efficacy in alleviating depressive symptoms among parents residing in low-resource rural communities.

Finally, Aaron and Chesley (2003) report on the positive spillover effects of improving health care providers' knowledge of the implications of lack of access to basic health care for maternal and child health for disparities in low birth weight between African American and European American clients, for which health care providers play a major role in their capacity to substantially reduce this gap. As these examples illustrate, these programs reduced health inequities by casting such efforts within a lifespan approach that connected personal development to ecological support and social structures. These are but a few examples of such efforts (see Williams et al., 2013, for a review of several more).

In bringing clarity about how disparities can be addressed and eliminated, it is important to note that, while there are clear and relatively consistent patterns of health advantages tied to economically and socially privileged ethnicities, there are many examples of poorer outcomes and more problematic pathways even for more advantaged groups (Braveman, 2014). The relation of social and economic privilege to health equity is not always uniform or straightforward. For example, males tend to have shorter lifespans than females, and breast cancer rates are similar for non-Hispanic European American and African American women but much higher for these two groups than for Hispanic, Asian, or Native

American women (Ward et al., 2004). This suggests that having privileged positions is not always protective and that the risk patterns are directly based on relative social status. The life-course approach, particularly because it can track the equifinality of multiple causal pathways (how different pathways can lead to similar health status) and multifinality (how similar dispositions and life-course experiences can lead to divergent outcomes), enables the disentanglement of more complicated patterns and uncovers opportunities for equity promotion (Braveman, 2006; Moy et al., 2005).

REGULATIONS, LAWS, AND LEGAL PRACTICES AFFECTING HEALTH EQUITIES

A second vector of great impact on health equity, in addition to sound lifespan as conceptualized by developmental science, comprises the regulations, policies, and laws regarding health rights, health access, and treatment and care (Rosenbaum et al., 2012). For instance, the linkages of discriminatory practices to inequity in criminal and civil laws have been well documented. Although these laws are not directly about health care, they can affect health opportunities, risk, and likely course (Satcher, 2001). The latter includes how differential treatment within the criminal justice system, access to affordable and sound housing, and opportunity to reside in communities with protection from environmental toxins and imminent and unpredictable threat to safety can all affect health.

The realm of legal/regulatory practices and policies has been often examined apart from life-course theory and biomedical research. There are a few instances in which legal and regulatory constraints or biases in practices are mentioned as contributing to health risk and disparities (Daniels et al., 2009; Sen, 2009). Conversely, the documentation of health-disparity patterns has been the impetus for numerous reviews of how legal ambiguities affect and perpetuate those disparities (Bobinski, 2003). Grounded within practices emanating from the civil rights movement, inequities in the applications or procedural manifestations of laws can provide a basis for legal efforts to change the laws, thereby requiring adherence to prescribed remedies or opportunities for changes in regulations or laws that impact health and health outcomes. However, examination of the regulatory and legal realm's role in health equity is relatively disconnected from the developmental and biomedical efforts that have been undertaken to address health disparities. Typically, the methods of analyses differ and do not readily translate across disciplines. That is, an integrative approach to address health equity that involves regulations and laws and biomedical and human development research is nonexistent.

Given that health disparities are both a life-course developmental issue and a legal/civil rights issue, there is great need to bring attention to ways regulations and laws affect developmental influences on health equity as well as ways access to healthy environments, supportive developmental settings, nondiscriminatory educational, employment, housing, and criminal justice and civil legal systems, and health knowledge and care promote healthier development or greater morbidity. This awareness should be given increased attention by those engaged in biomedical and developmental trajectory research in model formulations and population variation explanations. This suggestion implies that new empirical paradigms of science are needed to better understand and explain the impact, variation, and implication of laws on the health of individuals and groups most negatively affected by those laws and how laws and regulations may benefit healthy development (protection from risk, access to care) of some groups (Matthew, 2015). Moreover, experiments to test policies that are designed to eliminate disparities in practice efforts through changing regulations and laws need to be rigorously evaluated, with particular consideration given to those who are responsible for their implementation and how the regulations are applied. This kind of information, often ignored in studies of health disparities, could be useful in our efforts to facilitate health equity. As several authors have noted, there is need for deeper and sounder understanding of how laws and regulations at federal, state, and local levels create and constrain opportunities for equity; how implementation of those laws and regulations directs procedures toward or away from equity; the ways laws and regulations are integrated into health care management, patient education and empowerment, and training of practitioners toward equity; and how at patient–system contact these play out in affecting health disparities (Bobinski, 2003; Matthew, 2015). There are numerous opportunities to examine these inquiries empirically. For example, studies that have been conducted to examine the relation between regulations that promote health or impede health risk and health disparities (e.g., tobacco regulation), as well as those demonstrating differential effects by demographic and economic groups (Thomas et al., 2008), offer a model for our consideration.

In addition to aiding reconciliation of observations and conclusions from legal and scientific analyses, pursuit of empirical understanding of the impact of legal policies and procedures also can suggest opportunities for moving toward health equities (Matthew, 2015; Moy et al., 2005). For example, bias recognition training of health care providers may help reduce the difference in health care quality and use observed between minority and nonminority patients. Yet, economic and practice benchmarks such as patient satisfaction and relative reduction in overall health care costs may also promote this same outcome (Bobinski, 2003).

Findings from these studies can then be interpreted with consideration of how results can be translated to address life-course variations in health. This approach may uncover nuanced variations in needs, depending on the health care issue and the population facing disparities (Satcher, 2001).

As with lifespan-based developmental and biomedical research, there are examples from the literature that suggest points of opportunity to advance the health equity agenda (IOM, 2002). For example, the National Conference of State Legislatures lists numerous laws that were enacted in 2014 to reduce disparities, including regulations targeting provider bias finance inequities and differential patterns of health risk by gender and ethnic group (http://www.ncsl. org/research/health/2014-health-disparities-legislation.asp). However, almost all the efforts undertaken are being launched without a true scientific evaluation of the effects necessary to be validated as soundly scientific. Given the transformative financing, access, and methods of regulating health care that are in the Affordable Care Act, careful scientific tracking of how these strategies and approaches affect disparities (and perhaps more miniexperiments to determine the most beneficial policy and practices within the act's major tenets) seem likely to reveal important opportunities for major improvements regarding disparities.

In addition to an empirical focus on the impact of health systems–related laws and regulations on health equity, there is also the need for more robust and careful empirical delineation of indirect effects of other aspects of human life on health, such as housing, education, employment, and income, and how these are impacted by legal policies and practices that also affect health functioning. Such information is needed because empirical documentation is often limited to showing that groups facing racial and sex discrimination or who are subjected to housing in locations with environmental toxins, or overincluded and more harshly treated in the criminal justice system, have greater health risk and poorer outcomes. In most instances, there are multiple contributors and solutions to inequities. However, without more specific scientific analysis, only general suggestions are plausible.

Significant characterization of differential impacts of specific actions or practices in relation to these legal issues affecting health equity is almost absent from the literature (see IOM, 2002, and Williams et al., 2013, for a few examples that are exceptions). For example, how might improvements in legal protection provided to youth from lower economic and minority populations who are subjected to family violence affect their mental and physical health? Could consistent practices across all economic and ethnic groups reduce disparities? Systematic tracking, study of relation across variables, and sound experiments (randomized controlled trials or close variants) regarding legal system discriminatory laws and practices to formulate potential solutions for disparities are nonexistent. Policies and practices cascade through the lives of individuals and groups, having far-reaching impacts, without scientific study of the roles of laws and regulations in health equity to date. There is a grave need to document and understand how they impact health—this is an oversight in need of remediation.

SUMMARY AND CONCLUSIONS

In this chapter we present suggested directions in response to the question: *How central should health disparities/health equities be in the areas of health research, evaluation of accumulated research, advisement about practices, and policy suggestions?* We suggest that health equity should be paramount to such work. This contention is based on the notion that health equity is a fundamental form of justice emanating from basic human rights. Additionally, if it is not central in our efforts to address health disparities, it is very likely that, instead of expending effort to reduce inequities, attention will be focused on documenting the already-established fact that our society is grappling with large and serious disparities. Instead, we propose a shift to analyze what can be discerned about what will reduce inequities and what corrective actions can be taken.

We suggest two lines of inquiry and a method of organizing information in order to advance the agenda away from problem identification toward identifying solutions to determine what is studied about health equity, and how what is studied about health equity is conceptualized, analyzed, interpreted, and integrated into the larger field of research and application. The first step in this systematic inquiry is to cast the central role of health equity within a lifespan framework. This framework explicitly links the micro- and basic biological processes to more complex person, group, and societal patterns. Understanding these patterns is fundamental to understanding and addressing disparities. The second step is to apply the tools of scientific study to understanding the legal and political realm affecting disparities—the laws, regulations, practices, and implementation patterns that directly impact health and health care as well as the civil and criminal laws that epidemiological studies have linked to disparities (e.g., discrimination in criminal justice processing, violence in communities, and environmental toxin exposure). In addition to applying these two lines of scientific inquiry, to move beyond repeated documentation of disparities, a paradigm shift is needed to a primary focus on organizing, reviewing, and valuing scientific work based on how it is promising for reducing disparities and for revealing mechanisms and other empirical evidence that will move us toward health equity. The latter approach holds promise for relatively greater reliability and objectivity than most other methods, which suggests that together these two foci may have substantial promise toward health equities.

REFERENCES

Aaron, K. F., and F. D. Chesley, Jr. 2003. Beyond rhetoric: What we need to know to eliminate disparities. *Ethnicity and Disease* 13(3 Suppl. 3):9–11.

Acevedo-Garcia, D., T. L. Osypuk, R. E. Werbel, E. R. Meara, D. M. Cutler, and L. Berkman. 2004. Does housing mobility policy improve health? *Housing Policy Debate* 15:49–98.

APHA (American Public Health Association). 2015. *Better health through equity: Case studies in reframing public health work.* Available at https://www.apha.org/~/media/files/pdf/topics/equity/equity_stories.ashx.

Beach, S. R. H., S. M. Kogan, G. H. Brody, Y.-F. Chen, M. K. Lei, and V. M. Murry. 2008. Change in caregiver depression as a function of the Strong African American Families Program. *Journal of Family Psychology* 22(2):241–252.

Bobinski, M. A. 2003. Health disparities and the law: Wrongs in search of a right. *American Journal of Law and Medicine* 29(2–3):363–380.

Braveman, P. 2006. Health disparities and health equity: Concepts and measurement. *Annual Review of Public Health* 27:167–194.

Braveman, P. 2014. What are health disparities and health equity? We need to be clear. *Public Health Reports* 129(Suppl 2):5–8.

Braveman, P., and C. Barclay. 2009. Health disparities beginning in childhood: A life-course perspective. *Pediatrics* 124(Suppl 3):S163–S175.

Brody, G. H., S. M. Kogan, Y.-F. Chen, and V. M. Murry. 2008. Long-term effects of the Strong African American Families Program on youths' conduct problems. *Journal of Adolescent Health* 43:474–481.

Bronfenbrenner, U., and P. A. Morris. 2006. The bioecological model of human development. In *The handbook of child psychology, vol. 1: Theoretical models of human development.* Hoboken, NJ: Wiley, 793–828.

Daniels, N., B. Saloner, and A. Gelpi. Access, cost, and financing: Achieving an ethical health reform. *Health Affairs* 28(5):w909–w916.

Garcia Coll, C., G. Lamberty, R. Jenkins, H. P. McAdoo, K. Crnic, B. H. Wasik, and H. Vazquez Garcia. 1996. An integrative model for the study of developmental competencies in minority children. *Child Development* 67:1891–1914.

Halfon, N., and M. Hochstein. 2002. Life course health development: An integrated framework for developing health, policy, and research. *Milbank Quarterly* 80(3):433–479.

IOM (Institute of Medicine). 2002. *Unequal treatment: Confronting racial and ethnic disparities in health care.* Washington, DC: The National Academies Press.

Lerner, R. M. 2006. Developmental science, developmental systems, and contemporary theories of human development. In *The handbook of child psychology, vol. 1: Theoretical models of human development.* Hoboken, NJ: Wiley, 1–17.

Ludwig, J., L. Sanbonmatsu, L. Gennetian, E. Adam, G. Duncan, L. Katz, and T. McDade. 2011. Neighborhoods, obesity, and diabetes: A randomized social experiment. *New England Journal of Medicine* 365:1509–1519.

Ludwig, J., G. Duncan, L. Gennetian, L. Katz, R. Kessler, J. Kling, and L. Sanbonmatsu. 2012. Neighborhood effects on the long-term well-being of low-income adults. *Science* 337(6101):1505–1510.

Matthew, D. B. 2015. *Just medicine: A cure for racial inequality in American health care*. New York: New York University Press.

Moy, E., E. Dayton, and C. M. Clancy. 2005. Compiling the evidence: The National Healthcare Disparities Reports. *Health Affairs* 24(2):376–387.

Murry, V. M., G. H. Brody, L. McNair, Z. Luo, F. X. Gibbons, M. Gerrard, and T. A. Wills. 2005. Parental involvement promotes rural African American youths' self-pride and sexual self-concepts. *Journal of Marriage and Family* 67:627–642.

Murry, V., G. Brody, Y. Chen, S. Kogan, and A. Brown. 2010. Long-term effects of the Strong African American Families Program on youths' alcohol use. *Journal of Consulting and Clinical Psychology* 78(2):281–285.

Murry, V. M., L. D. McNair, S. S. Myers, Y. F. Chen, and G. H. Brody. 2014. Intervention induced changes in perceptions of parenting and risk opportunities among rural African Americans. *Journal of Child and Family Studies* 23(2):422–436.

NRC (National Research Council). 2004. *Eliminating health disparities: Measurement and data needs*. Washington, DC: The National Academies Press.

Olds, D. L., J. Eckenrode, C. R. Henderson, Jr., H. Kitzman, J. Powers, R. Cole, and D. Luckey. 1997. Long-term effects of home visitation on maternal life course and child abuse and neglect: 15-year follow-up of a randomized trial. *Journal of the American Medical Association* 278(8):637–643.

Politzer, R. M., J. Yoon, R. G. Hughes, J. Regan, and M. H. Gatson. 2001. Inequality in America: The contribution of health centers in reducing and disparities in access to care. *Medical Care Research and Review* 58(2):234–248.

Rosenbaum, S., D. M. Frankford, S. Law, and R. E. Rosenblatt. 2012. *Law and the American health care system*. St. Paul, MN: West Academic.

Satcher, D. 2001. Our commitment to eliminate racial and ethnic health disparities. *Yale Journal of Health Policy, Law, and Ethics* 1(1):1–14.

Seidel, R., P. Tolan, V. M. Murry, and A. Diaz. 2016. Philosophical perspectives on social justice: A framework for discussing children, youth, and families health policy and research agenda. *NAM Perspectives*. Discussion Paper, National Academy of Medicine, Washington, DC.

Sen, A. 1999. *Development as freedom*. New York: Oxford University Press.

Sen, A. 2009. *The idea of justice*. Cambridge, MA: Belknap Press.

Shanahan, M. J., and J. D. Boardman. 2009. Genetics and behavior in the life course: A promising frontier. In *The craft of life course research*. New York: Guilford Press, 215–235.

Thomas S., D. Fayter, K. Misso, D. Ogilvie, M. Petticrew, M. Sowden, and G. Worthy. 2008. Population tobacco control interventions and their effects on social inequalities in smoking: Systematic review. *Tobacco Control* 17(4):230–237.

Tolan, P. H., D. H. Henry, D. Gorman-Smith, and M. Schoeny. 2016. *Family support at elementary school entry prevents adolescent violence*. Unpublished manuscript, University of Virginia, Charlottesville, VA.

Ward, E., A. Jemal, V. Cokkinides, G. K. Singh, C. Cardinez, A. Ghafoor, and M. Thun. 2004. Cancer disparities by race/ethnicity and socioeconomic status. *CA: A Cancer Journal for Clinicians* 54:78–93.

Whitehead, M. 1992. The concepts and principles of equity and health. *International Journal of Health Services* 22(3):429–445.

Williams, D. R., A. Selina, and S. Mohammed. 2013. Racism and health, I: Pathways and scientific evidence. *American Behavioral Scientist* 57(8):1152–1173.

3

THE CHARACTER ASSASSINATION OF BLACK MALES: SOME CONSEQUENCES FOR RESEARCH IN PUBLIC HEALTH

Alford A. Young Jr., PhD

A consequence of pervasive social inequality is the regard by those of higher socioeconomic standing of those at the bottom of American social hierarchies, especially men and boys of color, as unworthy citizens. In exploring the associations that Americans have made throughout history between poverty and unworthiness, historian Michael B. Katz (2013) has argued that many Americans have consistently maintained that people in poverty have brought that condition upon themselves, thus making them unworthy of public sympathy and support. Furthermore, Katz has documented that many believe that the poor have brought their condition upon themselves as a consequence of being embedded in moral, cultural, and biological deficiencies.

Being perceived as unworthy has powerful social consequences. Unworthiness fosters social undesirability, which, in turn, affects social interaction. This amounts to more than generating inner feelings of disdain among those in poverty or simply being looked upon with consternation by those with privilege. Instead, interaction with unworthy people often falls outside of the parameters of the codes of conduct and evaluative schemes that are applied to interactions with those deemed as worthy. Commonly embraced standards of fairness, justice, and appropriateness that are usually applied in the course of engaging others are drastically reconstituted during encounters with the socially undesirable. As a consequence, those deemed unworthy have very different—and often very disappointing—experiences in the societal institutions and spheres (e.g., schools, the workplace) that anchor everyday life. This experience constitutes the social situation of many African American males in contemporary society.

For men and boys of color, especially those who are socioeconomically disadvantaged, social unworthiness is rooted in their being portrayed as distinctively morally and culturally flawed (Anderson, 1990, 1999; Auletta, 1982; Billson, 1996; Liebow, 1967; Majors and Billson, 1992; Tolleson, 1997; Venkatesh, 2000, 2006; Wilson, 1987, 1992; Young, 2004). As this research has shown, these males register in the minds of the American public as threatening, hostile, aggressive, unconscientious, and incorrigible. Beliefs about their moral and cultural short-comings help engineer a warped vision of not only their capacities for positive individual and collective action but also of their very public identities. Hence, it is not simply what these individuals do as societal actors, but who they are that constitutes their problematic status in civil society. In other words, the very image of the black male body often conjures up indictment. Bearing the mark of unworthiness and the accompanying social undesirability that comes from it subjects African American males to an extreme form of *character assassination.*

A character assassination is an act of consistently presenting false or indicting arguments about a person in order to encourage his or her public dislike or mistrust. This effort can also take the form of slandering of a person with the intention of destroying public confidence in him or her (*Merriam-Webster*, 2015; for a more sociologically informed account, see Seidman, 2013). As a consequence of the emergence of the age of the underclass in late 20th-century America (occurring from the early 1980s through the end of the 20th century), African American males have been subjected to a character assassination that largely has to do with the public's increased sense of fear and anxiety about the urban landscape and its inhabitants throughout that time (Katz, 2013; Ralph and Chance, 2014; Russell-Brown, 2009; Venkatesh, 2000, 2006; Wacquant, 2001, 2005, 2010; Wilson, 1987; Young, 2004). As the concept of underclass has gained purchase as a mechanism for labeling socioeconomically marginalized, urban-based people of color over the past several decades, these individuals have been subjected to extremely negative readings of their social behavior and their dispositions. They also have been assumed to maintain flawed and fatalistic social outlooks. Often, these accounts are presumptions rather than directly informed understandings, because the external parties that make them do not necessarily have access to the inner feeling and beliefs of black males. Rather than coming from intimate knowledge about them, these accounts of their outlook are constituted from the images construed about their behaviors and public identities (Young, 2004).

Essentially, the character assassination of black males is an effect of longstanding implicit bias directed toward them. This bias, consisting of attitudes and stereotypes that shape understandings, behaviors, and decisions made about them, is done unconsciously and activated involuntarily (Blair, 2002; Rudman, 2004). Although implicit bias can involve both favorable and unfavorable assessments, it is obviously the unfavorable that are of concern here. What makes implicit bias so powerful is that it is not easily accessible through introspection or immediate self-reflection (Beattie, 2013; Kang et al., 2012). Hence, it is powerfully pervasive because it is so seamlessly woven into the everyday thinking of its holders (Eberhardt and Goff, 2005; Eberhardt et al., 2004; Goff et al., 2008a,b).

There is much recent evidence affirming how black male bodies are both thought about and engaged in ways that reflect character assassination and the implicit bias that circumscribes it. One form is the public conversations about the spate of black-male killings occurring at the hands of police officers and others claiming to act on behalf of justice. For example, after the killing of Trayvon Martin became public news, questions abounded as to whether he was a marijuana user and a petty criminal in the years prior to his February 2012 encounter with his killer, George Zimmerman (Alcindor, 2012; Alvarez, 2013; Robles, 2012). Furthermore, news of the killing of Michael Brown in Ferguson, Missouri, in August 2014 was followed by discussion of whether he was threateningly hostile and menacing to those he encountered immediately prior to his being shot and left dead in the streets of that St. Louis suburb (Alcindor et al., 2014; Tacopino, 2014).

Moreover, the public image associated with Tamir Rice—killed on November 22, 2014, in Cleveland by a police officer who came upon him as he was in possession of a toy gun—was that of a black male who appeared to the police as primed to do harm even as seemingly unconcerned African American children and adults shared space with him in a public park near the site of his killing (Fitzsimmons, 2014). Finally, there is the portrait of Freddie Gray—a 25-year-old ex-offender who died on April 19, 2015, after being shackled and placed without a seat belt in a Baltimore City police van. In some of the media coverage of this event and the subsequent court trial of the police officers indicted for Gray's death, he was referred to as the son of an illiterate heroin addict (Husband, 2015). These circumstances associated with deaths resemble those of many other African American males killed in recent years by police officers or law-enforcement officials, including Laquan McDonald (Ford, 2014), Quintonio LeGrier (Meisner, 2016), Jamar Clark (Pelissero, 2016; Walsh and Jany, 2015), Walter Scott (Elmore and MacDougall, 2015), Keith Lamont Scott (Fausset and Alcindor, 2016; Marusak and Washburn, 2016), Terence Crutcher (Vicent and Jones, 2016), Tyre King (Felton, 2016), Philando Castile (Sole and Wannarka, 2016), and Alton Sterling (Litten, 2016; Sanburn, 2016).

Media coverage of the public debate following the deaths of these and other African American males centered on two forms of public response and inquiry. One was whether these individuals conducted themselves as proper or deserving people. The other was whether they appeared to be highly threatening or dangerous in the moments prior to their deaths. In the course of these considerations, attention was devoted to whether each was a substance abuser, general delinquent, or an otherwise problematic person. Consequently, underlying the discourse from those who defend or otherwise try to validate the actions of those who killed these young men is the image of black males as badly behaved individuals who are threatening in and to American society. Implicit in these and other tragic deaths of such males was the notion that what they did, who they were, or how they appeared to be at the time in which they were approached by those who encountered them was credible explanation, if not complete justification, for what transpired. In short, the kind of discussions following what occurred to each individual reflects the most extreme form of character assassination—the devaluation of black male bodies.

More important, this portrait of African American males has been sustained by a barrage of negative images about them emanating from mainstream and social media (Altheide, 2002; Burgess et al., 2011; Chiricos and Eschholz, 2002; Dill and Burgess, 2012; Dixon, 2008; Dixon and Linz, 2000; Ellis et al., 2015; Entman and Rojecki, 2001; Ford, 1997, Jacobs, 2014; Kellstedt, 2003; Oliver, 2003; Oliver and Fonash, 2002; Opportunity Agenda, 2012). Such outlets are key mechanisms for fueling the negative public sentiment about black males. Through them, consistent images have been disseminated that reify the image of these males as unlawful, threatening, or unworthy.

Of course, that some of the black males have done terrible things to themselves as well as to other people cannot be dismissed or denied. Research on low-income, African American males has provided ample evidence that those who have ventured into these activities are conscious of what they have done and the societal impact that it has had (Harding, 2010; Sullivan, 1989; Venkatesh, 2000, 2006; Williams, 1989; Young, 2004). However, the depiction of these males as having the capacity to be self-reflective or conscientious is suppressed by the pervasiveness of the character assassination.

More critically, African American males who do nothing to contribute to the indicting public portrait of them suffer the consequences of this pervasive public portrait, as they are assumed to be as problematic as those who effectively contribute to it (Pager, 2007; Pager et al., 2009a, b; Quillian and Pager, 2001; Wacquant, 2001, 2005, 2010). These males experience everyday life and the social institutions that comprise it while being continually susceptible to a negative public identity that they in no way have helped to sustain. This being the case, there is much work to be done to reconstitute the character of African American males that extends far beyond any superficial or shortsighted mandate for them to desist from engaging in problematic behavior. That work involves a more thorough assessment of the effects of black-male character assassination through a public health lens and then encouraging societal change to eradicate it. This effort necessarily extends beyond the (still necessary) effort to challenge and remediate the conduct of the police and other agents of authority, as they, too, often function with impunity with regard to black males.

CONTENDING WITH THE EFFECTS OF THE CHARACTER ASSASSINATION

The character assassination of black males often compels them to respond in ways that reflect a *stereotype threat,* which is a manifestation of implicit bias. This threat is a situational predicament in which individuals are or feel themselves to be at risk of confirming negative stereotypes about a social group in which they hold membership (Inzlicht and Schmader, 2011; Shih et al., 2011). Such threat most often has been investigated as a factor for the lower performance of African Americans on the standardized tests used for college admissions (Steele and Aronson, 1995). In such cases, the argument has been that such individuals perform poorly on such tests when conscious of the belief that others regard them as less capable of performing well. It is important to acknowledge that an individual must not necessarily subscribe to the stereotype for it to be activated. Instead, performance anxiety is activated by the stereotype in that its existence depletes the working memory of individuals. Consequently, rather than drawing on the relevant information, understandings, skill sets, or efficacies for task completion, individuals are distracted by the anxiety from performing most effectively (Beilock et al., 2007).

Stereotype threat is applicable only to those who generally perform well. Accordingly, its conceptual value rests in the effort to discern the bases for the less-than-optimal performance of people who are traditionally high performers (Steele, 2010). Introducing the concept of stereotype threat here, however, allows space for considering how threat based on a stereotype can stymie the agency of people irrespective of how highly they may perform at certain tasks or how enriched their skill sets may be for navigating everyday life. The threat for black males, then, is that, irrespective of their class status or ability to access societal resources, they must confront a threat—an assassinated character—that is deeply rooted in flawed, stereotypical depictions of such individuals (more will be said later about the relevance of socioeconomic class differences for addressing the character assassination of these males).

Moreover, stereotype threat is an explicitly psychological phenomenon. However, the point here is not to psychologize the consequences of the character assassination of black males. Instead, it is to draw attention to how such a negative generalized public portrait can bear upon the everyday lives of individuals who are subjected to it, thus drawing attention to the sociological dimensions of the threat.

The major effect of the character assassination of black males, aside from exposure to the kinds of physical assaults documented earlier, is the proliferation of trauma. In public health studies, various approaches have unfolded for researching trauma in the lives of African American males. Traditional approaches involve researching the psychological and physiological consequences of witnessing or experiencing physical assault and explicit violence (Prothrow-Stith, 1991; Ralph, 2014). This effort has been supplemented with studies that explore how various stimuli aside from exposure to violence affect the emotional and physiological well-being of African American males (Brown et al., 2000; Ellis et al., 2015; Griffith, 2015; Griffith et al., 2012, 2015; Watkins, et al., 2010; Williams and Collins, 1995). Schools, workplaces, and other institutional settings have been the focal points for some of these studies. Indeed, another arena of public health research on African American males has centered more specifically on the health and well-being outcomes emanating from perceived experiences with racism. Here, sociologists such as David Williams, Chaquita Collins, and Tony Brown, among others, have shown that the health consequences of racism include various forms of trauma which affect the psychological and physiological states of being of these males (Brown et al., 2000; Williams and Collins, 1995).

Without question, these more traditional inquiries must continue. However, there is more work to be done aside from addressing the psychological and physiological consequences of these phenomena. Is it shortsighted to assume that the terrain for public health inquiry concerning black males be restricted to how they respond to the prevalence of violence and threats to physical well-being or to perceptions of explicit racism in their lives? While it is imperative that such work continue, it is equally so that the public health agenda expand to include investigation of the psychological and sociological effects of living in a social world circumscribed by imagery that constitutes African American males as hostile, aggressive, and incapable of self-regulating behavior. Indeed, more thorough considerations may allow for a better grasp of the range of trauma that may be produced from living under the conditions of character assassination. Hence, more critical attention must be given to how black males take account of and respond to the broad range of conditions and circumstances that pertain to the character assassination. This effort involves further unpacking the social-psychological, psychological, or physiological ramifications that may exist for males who continually engage a social world that sustains their character assassination.

That black males often believe that they must exemplify or validate various kinds of vulgar or rugged masculinities that have been associated with them, even if they do not personally adhere to these depictions, has been well documented in social-scientific inquiry (Ford, 2008, 2011; Hooks, 2003; Hunter and Davis, 1992). Their doing so often appears to them as a prerequisite for attaining the social and physical security necessary to engage everyday life in turbulent communities (Anderson, 1990; Ford, 2011; Majors and Billson, 1992). It is also the case that black men consistently wrestle with the persistence of the imagery tied to vulgar or rugged masculinities as these men think about what kinds of self-images to foster in their social and intimate interactions (Hooks, 2003; Neal, 2006, 2013). This circumstance is a precursor to the issue raised here in that, in addition to having to situate oneself against the traditional vulgar or rugged masculinities associated with black men, these individuals must also situate themselves against the imagery associated with the character assassination.

In the domain of public health research, however, the concern rests not in how males manage social interaction in public spaces but rather in devising means and measures to assess any individual and collective emotional impact of consistent subjection to character assassination. The existence of character assassination may not result in any explicit impingement upon individual behavior or conduct. However, the extreme surveillance of and critical social judgment made about the conduct, action, or disposition exemplified by black males may be causal factors for a range of unhealthy emotional and physical states of being.

THE CALL FOR NEW SCHOLARSHIP IN PUBLIC HEALTH

Black males are continually forced to take regard of the narrow parameters by which others interpret and respond to their public behavior. Ultimately, this results in a stultification of their agency. Hence, it is imperative that focused attention be given to the personal effect of everyday living in a state of social unworthiness. While the work of the public health scholars cited earlier provides evidence that much of black-male agency with regard to dietary practices and social activities poses threats to their physical well-being (hypertension, anxiety, and other conditions aside from those that subject them to violence), there still remains the issue of how living as a black male, coupled with how continual reflection on how oneself is being interpreted by others as a black male, may cause threats to or problems with one's personal health and well-being.

The new agenda in public health research must involve broadening the scope of understanding of what is at stake for African American males, given the construction of the character assassination. That is, it must involve documenting and interpreting the effects of basic, everyday living under that lens for these males. Part of this effort involves studying the psychological and physiological effects of engaging police and other agents of authority. It also means exploring more deeply how black males feel about their schooling experiences in terms of how they believe they are depicted by their teachers, principals, and other school officials. Furthermore, it means gauging how men react to their employment situations, including the personal effects of contending with the reactions and responses of actual and potential coworkers and employers.

Of course, black males have access to different resources for managing and interpreting these and other experiences. Their particular class standing is an indicator of the material, emotional, cultural, and cognitive resources at their disposal for dealing with them. Hence, it is important to assess the impact of character assassination not simply for males who are highly marginalized, and thus most likely to experience the extremely negative consequences of the character assassination, but also for males who experience it while in possession of higher educational degrees, white-collar jobs, or the material means to purchase resources to counteract the effects of the character assassination. Implicit here is that the men who may seem most removed from the negative public portraits of black men also have to engage everyday life with those portraits as backdrop to public interpretations of their behaviors and dispositions.

In short, this agenda must involve inquiry into how black males feel about flawed public assertions about black masculinity and social constructions of black-male identity and the investigation of the bearing this has on their physical and emotional well-being across differences in class, status, and social location. The ways these constructions are formed remain the purview of many standard social science fields of inquiry (e.g., sociology, psychology, and communication studies). Precise understanding of their effects on these males, however, is the property of public health studies.

Inclusive in this effort is the need to be open and accepting of the notion that black males are vulnerable people rather than just victimizers. Obviously, some black males are the latter, but all must be seen as the former, that is, as socially insecure, questioning of themselves, and threatened, rather than simply as purveyors of threat and insecurity foisted upon others (Collins, 2004; Franklin, 1984, 1994). The effects of their being insecure, questioning, and threatened, especially as victims of character assassination, is particularly important to explore as a public health matter.

To most appropriately support this effort, however, an alternative public vision of black males also must come into being. It must capture more accurately and thoroughly how these males envision social opportunity and the barriers that they perceive. Aside from the general mandate of reenvisioning black males as more complex than is provided by the imagery resulting from character assassination, there is a more direct mandate for those in and interested in public health. This involves advancing new and robust arguments about what constitutes healthy masculinity with regard to black males.

CONCLUSION: DEMYSTIFYING THE CHARACTER OF BLACK MALES

The absence of broader public awareness and acceptance of an alternative image of black males means that the enduring image is one of males who are presumed to be unable to function in any measured and conscientious manner. Thus, they are falsely understood to be preoccupied with living for the present and with reactive rather than deliberative ways of dealing with the circumstances in their lives and with other people. The portrait readily facilitates a sustained vision of these males as fatalistic in social outlook and behavior. Ultimately, any wholesale mitigation of the character assassination of these males can occur only if there is a shift in the public imagination of them.

An effort to demystify the character of black males must first involve acknowledging that fatalism is an incomplete conceptual scheme for encapsulating the social outlooks of the racialized poor (Rios, 2011; Venkatesh, 2000, 2006; Young, 2004). These studies and others (Fergus et al., 2014; Noguera, 2008; Wilson, 1996; Young, 2004) indicate that black males do not necessarily reject mainstream institutional spheres such as schooling but rather have negative experiences with individuals in these spheres. The result is that they face problems with their encounters with schools, employers, and legal authorities such as the police, but not with schooling, employment, or the institution of law in a general sense. Research reveals that such males do value schools, jobs, and family; yet they struggle with their personal experiences in each of these and other domains (Lewis-McCoy, 2014; Noguera, 2008; Venkatesh, 2006; Wilson, 1996; Young, 2004). Hence, it is too simple to regard this population as engulfed in thinking that the world is against them and that they react with aggression and hostility because they believe there is nothing that they can do to change these conditions.

The ensuing challenge for researchers and interested parties, then, is to re-envision black males as complex human beings—a mixture of socially defined positive and negative attributes, much like other people—rather than wholly unworthy. It means embracing a vision of them as adherents to the same cultural schemas that apply to many Americans—as committed to the value of family, education, employment, and socioeconomic opportunity—even if actions sometimes surface due to the denial of the capacity to access these desires and outcomes. It means that the existence of black males in trouble or who are troubling should not be the bedrock for interpreting the character and dispositions of all such males, nor should it be the basis for a default depiction of black males as inherently flawed people. For the sake of black males, the effects of their character assassination mandates further, more intense, and more specific forms of study. However, the public acknowledgment and acceptance of an alternative image of black males and black masculinity requires work alongside that of public health scholars, and this work necessarily involves the rest of us who function outside of the formal arena of public health studies.

REFERENCES

Alcindor, Y. 2012. Trayvon Martin: Typical teen or troublemaker? *USA Today,* December 11.

Alcindor, Y., M. Bello, and A. Madhani. 2014. Chief: Officer noticed Brown carrying suspected stolen cigars. *USA Today,* August 15.

Altheide, D. 2002. *Creating fear: News and the construction of crisis.* New York: Aldine Transaction.

Alvarez, L. 2013. Defense in Trayvon Martin case raises questions about the victim's character. *New York Times,* May 23.

Anderson, E. 1990. *Streetwise: Race, class, and change in an urban community.* Chicago: University of Chicago Press.

Anderson, E. 1999. *Code of the street: Decency, violence, and the moral life of the inner city.* New York: Norton.

Auletta, K. 1982. *The underclass.* New York: Random House.

Beattie, G. 2013. *Our racist heart? An exploration of unconscious prejudice in everyday life.* London: Routledge.

Beilock, S. L., R. J. Rydell, and A. R. McConnell. 2007. Stereotype threat and working memory: Mechanisms, alleviation, and spillover. *Journal of Experimental Psychology: General* 136(2):256–276.

Billson, J. M. 1996. *Pathways to manhood: Young black males struggle for identity.* Piscataway, NJ: Transaction.

Blair, I. V. 2002. The malleability of automatic stereotypes and prejudice. *Personality and Social Psychology Review* 6(3):242–261.

Brown, T. N., D. R. Williams, J. S. Jackson, H. W. Neighbors, M. Torres, S. L. Sellers, and K. T. Brown. 2000. Being black and feeling blue: The mental-health consequences of racial discrimination. *Race & Society* 2(2):117–131.

Burgess, M. C., K. E. Dill, S. P. Stermer, S. R. Burgess, and B. P. Brown. 2011. Playing with prejudice: The prevalence and consequences of racial stereotypes in video games. *Media Psychology* 14:289–311.

Chiricos, T., and S. Eschholz. 2002. The racial and ethnic typification of crime and the criminal typification of race and ethnicity in local television news. *Journal of Research in Crime and Delinquency* 39:400–420.

Collins, P. H. 2004. *Black sexual politics: African Americans, gender, and the new racism.* New York: Routledge.

Dill, K. E., and M. C. R. Burgess. 2012. Influence of black masculinity game exemplars on social judgments. *Simulation & Gaming* 44(4):562–585.

Dixon, T. 2008. Network news and racial beliefs: Exploring the connection between national television news exposure and stereotypical perceptions of African Americans. *Journal of Communication* 58(2):321–337.

Dixon, T. L., and D. Linz. 2000. Over-representation and under-representation of African Americans and Latinos as lawbreakers on television news. *Journal of Communication* 50(2):131–154.

Eberhardt, J. L., and P. A. Goff. 2005. Seeing race. In *Social psychology of prejudice: Historical and contemporary issues,* edited by C. S. Crandall and M. Schaller. Seattle, WA: Lewinian Press. Pp. 163–183.

Eberhardt, J. L., P. A. Goff, V. J. Purdie, and P. G. Davies. 2004. Seeing black: Race, representation, and visual perception. *Journal of Personality and Social Psychology* 87:876–893.

Ellis, K. R., D. M. Griffith, J. O. Allen, R. J. Thorpe Jr., and M. A. Bruce. 2015. If you do nothing about stress, the next thing you know, you're shattered: Perspectives on African American men's stress, coping, and health from African American men and key women in their lives. *Social Science & Medicine* 139:107–114.

Elmore, C., and D. MacDougall. 2015. Man shot and killed by North Charleston police officer after traffic stop; SLED investigating. *Post and Courier,* April 4. Available from http://www.postandcourier.com/article/20150404/PC16/150409635.

Entman, R. M., and A. Rojecki. 2001. *The black image in the white mind: Media and race in America.* Chicago: University of Chicago Press.

Fausset, R., and Y. Alcindor. 2016. Video by wife of Keith Scott shows her pleas to police. *New York Times,* September 23. Available from http://www.nytimes.com/2016/09/24/us/charlotte-keith-scott-shooting-video.html.

Felton, R. 2016. "Our kids can't play with toy guns": Tyre King police shooting a painful reminder. *The Guardian,* September 20. Available from https://www.theguardian.com/us-news/2016/sep/20/tyre-king-columbus-ohio-police-shooting.

Fergus, E., P. Noguera, and M. Martin. 2014. *Schooling for resilience: Improving the life trajectories of African American and Latino males.* Cambridge, MA: Harvard Education Press.

Fitzsimmons, E. 2014. 12-year-old boy dies after police in Cleveland shoot him. *New York Times,* November 23.

Ford, K. 2008. Gazing into the distorted looking glass: Masculinity, femininity, appearance ideals, and the black body. *Sociology Compass* 2(3):1096–1114.

Ford, K. 2011. Doing fake masculinity, being real men: Present and future constructions of self among black college men. *Symbolic Interaction* 34(1):38–62.

Ford, Q. 2014. Cops: Boy, 17, fatally shot by officer after refusing to drop knife. *Chicago Tribune,* October 21. Available from http://www.chicagotribune.com/news/local/breaking/chi-chicago-shootings-violence-20141021-story.html.

Ford, T. E. 1997. Effects of stereotypical television portrayals of African Americans on person perception. *Social Psychology Quarterly* 60:266–278.

Franklin, C. W. 1984. *The changing definition of masculinity.* New York: Plenum Press.

Franklin, C. W. 1994. Ain't I a man? The efficacy of black masculinities for men's studies in the 1990s. In *The American black male: His present status and his future,* edited by R. G. Majors and J. U. Gordon. Chicago: Nelson-Hall. Pp. 271–284.

Goff, P. A., J. L. Eberhardt, M. Williams, and M. C. Jackson. 2008a. Not yet human: Implicit knowledge, historical dehumanization, and contemporary consequences. *Journal of Personality and Social Psychology* 94:292–306.

Goff, P. A., C. M. Steele, and P. G. Davies. 2008b. The space between us: Stereotype threat and distance in interracial contexts. *Journal of Personality and Social Psychology* 94:91–107.

Griffith, D. M. 2015. "I AM a man": Manhood, minority men's health and health equity. *Ethnicity & Disease* 25(3):287–293.

Griffith, D. M., K. E. Gunter, and D. C. Watkins. 2012. Measuring masculinity in research on men of color: Findings and future directions. *American Journal of Public Health* 102:S187–S194.

Griffith, D. M., L. Brinkley-Rubinstein, M. A. Bruce, R. J. Thorpe Jr., and J. M. Metzl. 2015. The interdependence of African American men's definitions of manhood and health. *Family and Community Health* 38(4):284–296.

Harding, D. J. 2010. *Living the drama: Community, conflict, and culture among inner-city boys.* Chicago: University of Chicago Press.

Hooks, B. 2003. *We real cool: Black men and masculinity.* New York: Routledge.

Hunter, A. G., and J. E. Davis. 1992. Constructing gender: An exploration of Afro-American men's conceptualization of manhood. *Gender & Society* 6(3):464–479.

Husband, A. 2015. CNN describes Freddie Gray as "son of an illiterate heroin addict," Twitter goes nuts. *MEDIAite,* November 30. Available from http://www. mediaite.com/online/ cnn-describes-freddie-gray-as-son-of-an-illiterate-heroin-addict-twitter-goes-nuts.

Inzlicht, M., and T. Schmader, eds. 2011. *Stereotype threat: Theory, process, and application.* New York: Oxford University Press. P. 5.

Jacobs, R. N. 2014. Media sociology and the study of race. In *Media sociology: A reappraisal,* edited by S. Waisbord. Malden, MA: Polity. Pp. 168–187.

Kang, J., M. Bennett, D. Carbado, P. Casey, N. Dasgupta, D. Faigman, R. Godsil, A. G. Greenwald, J. Levinson, and J. Mnookin. 2012. Implicit bias in the courtroom. *UCLA Law Review* 59:1126–1186.

Katz, M. B. 2013. *The undeserving poor: America's enduring confrontation with poverty,* 2nd Ed. New York: Oxford University Press.

Kellstedt, P. M. 2003. *The mass media and the dynamics of American racial attitudes.* Cambridge, UK: Cambridge University Press.

Lewis-McCoy, R. L. 2014. *Inequality in the promised land: Race, resources and suburban schooling.* Stanford, CA: Stanford University Press.

Liebow, E. 1967. *Tally's Corner: A study of Negro streetcorner men.* Boston: Little, Brown.

Litten, K. 2016. Alton Sterling shooting death: What we know so far. *Times Picayune,* July 6. Available from http//www.nola.com/politics/index.ssf/2016/07/alton_ sterling_what_we_know.html.

Majors, R., and J. M. Billson. 1992. *Cool pose: The dilemmas of black manhood in America.* New York: Lexington Books.

Marmot, M., S. Friel, R. Bell, T. A. J. Houweling, and S. Taylor. 2008. Closing the gap in a generation: Health equity through action on the social determinants of health. *Lancet* 372:166-1669.

Marusak, J., and M. Washburn. 2016. CMPD releases full video of fatal Keith Lamont Scott shooting. *Charlotte Observer,* October 4. Available from http://www.charlotteob-server.com/news/special- reports/charlotte-shooting-protests/article105978672.html.

Meisner, J. 2016. Texts using version of N-word at issue in LeGrier police shooting. *Chicago Tribune,* July 14. Available from http//www.chicagotribune.com/news/local/breaking/ct-quintonio-legrier-bettie-jones-texts-met-20160714-story.html.

Merriam-Webster, Inc. 2015. Character assassination. Available from http://www.merriam-webster.com/ dictionary/character%20assassination.

Neal, M. A. 2006. *New black man.* New York: Routledge.

Neal, M. A. 2013. *Looking for Leroy: Illegible black masculinities.* New York: New York University Press.

Noguera, P. A. 2008. *The trouble with black boys and other reflections on race, equity, and the future of public education.* New York: John Wiley & Sons.

Oliver, M. B. 2003. African American men as "criminal and dangerous": Implications of media portrayals of crime on the "criminalization" of African American men. *Journal of African American Studies* 7(2):3–18.

Oliver, M. B., and D. Fonash. 2002. Race and crime in the news: Whites' identification and misidentification of violent and nonviolent criminal suspects. *Media Psychology* 4(2):137–156.

Opportunity Agenda. 2012. *Social science literature review: Media representations and impact on the lives of black men and boys.* Available from http://opportunityagenda.org/literature_review_media_representations_and_impact_lives_black_men_and_boys.

Pager, D. 2007. *Marked: Race, crime, and finding work in an era of mass incarceration.* Chicago, IL: University of Chicago Press.

Pager, D., B. Western, and B. Bonikowski. 2009a. Discrimination in a low-wage labor market: A field experiment. *American Sociological Review* 74(5):777–799.

Pager, D., B. Western, and N. Sugie. 2009b. Sequencing disadvantage: Barriers to employment facing young black and white men with criminal records. *Annals of the American Academy of Political and Social Science* 623:195–213.

Pelissero, S. 2016. Cops won't be charged in death of black Minn. man. *USA Today,* March 30. Available from http://www.usatoday.com/story/news/nation/2016/03/30/officers-wont-charged-jamar-clarks-death/82462624/.

Prothrow-Stith, D. 1991. *Deadly consequences: How violence is destroying our teenage population and a plan to begin solving the problem.* New York: HarperCollins.

Quillian, L. G., and Pager, D. 2001. Black neighborhoods, higher crime? The role of racial stereotypes in evaluations of neighborhood crime. *American Journal of Sociology* 107(3):717–767.

Ralph, L. 2014. *Renegade dreams: Living through injury in gangland Chicago.* Chicago, IL: University of Chicago Press.

Ralph, L., and K. Chance. 2014. Legacies of fear. *Transition* 133:137–143.

Rios, V. 2011. Punished: Policing the lives of black and Latino boys. New York: NYU Press.

Robles, F. 2012. Multiple suspensions paint complicated portrait of Trayvon Martin. *Miami Herald*, March 26.

Rudman, L. A. 2004. Social justice in our minds, homes, and society: The nature, causes, and consequences of implicit bias. *Social Justice Research* 17(2):129–142.

Russell-Brown, K. 2009. *The color of crime*. New York: NYU Press.

Sanburn, J. 2016. Alton sterling is one of more than 100 black men killed by police in 2016. *Time*, July 6. Available from http://time.com/4394802/alton-sterling-police-shooting-baton-rouge.

Seidman, S. 2013. Defilement and disgust: Theorizing the other. *American Journal of Cultural Sociology* 1(1):3–25.

Shih, M. J., T. L. Pittinsky, and G. C. Ho. 2011. Stereotype boost: Positive outcomes from the activation of positive stereotypes. In *Stereotype threat: Theory, process, and application*, edited by M. Inzlicht and T. Schmader. New York: Oxford University Press. Pp. 141–143.

Sole, J., and R. Wannarka. 2016. Philando Castille decision: Choi must not repeat Freeman's missteps. *StarTribune*, October 7. Available from http://www.startribune.com/philandocastille-decision-choi-must-not-repeat-freeman-s-missteps/396364161.

Steele, C. M. 2010. *Whistling Vivaldi: How stereotypes affect us and what we can do*. New York: W.W. Norton.

Steele, C. M., and J. Aronson. 1995. Stereotype threat and the intellectual test performance of African Americans. *Journal of Personality and Social Psychology* 69(5):797–811

Sullivan, M. 1989. *Getting paid: Youth crime and work in the inner city*. Ithaca, NY: Cornell University Press.

Tacopino, J. 2014. Darren Wilson on why he shot Michael Brown. *New York Post*, November 25.

Tolleson, J. 1997. Death and transformation: The reparative power of violence in the lives of young black inner-city gang members. *Smith College Studies in Social Work* 67(3):415–431.

Venkatesh, S. A. 2000. *American project: The rise and fall of a modern ghetto*. Cambridge, MA: Harvard University Press.

Venkatesh, S. 2006. *Off the books: The underground economy of the urban poor*. Cambridge, MA: Harvard University Press.

Vicent, S., and C. Jones. 2016. Tulsa police chief on fatal shooting of Terence Crutcher: "There was no gun." *Tulsa World*, September 20. Available from http://www.tulsa-world.com/news/local/tulsa-police-chief-on-fatal-shooting-of-terence-crutcher-there/article_198d5656-bfbe-5a6d-b108-53c6d304be9e.html.

Wacquant, L. 2001. Deadly symbiosis: When ghetto and prison meet and mesh. *Punishment and Society* 3:95–133.

Wacquant, L. 2005. Race as civil felony. *International Social Science Journal* 57(183):127–142.

Wacquant, L. 2010. Class, race, and hyperincarceration in revanchist America. *Daedalus* 139:74–90.

Walsh, P., and L. Jany. 2015. Anger builds after police shoot assault suspect in Minneapolis. *StarTribune*, November 16. Available From http://www. startribune.

com/police-officer-shoots-north-minneapolis-assault-suspect-during-physical-struggle/349730171.

Watkins, D. C., R. L. Walker, and D. M. Griffith. 2010. Meta-study of black male mental health and well-being. *Journal of Black Psychology* 36(3):303–330.

Williams, D. R., and C. Collins. 1995. US socioeconomic and racial differences in health: Patterns and explanations. *Annual Review of Sociology* 21:349–386.

Williams, T. 1989. *Cocaine kids: The inside story of a teenage drug ring.* New York: De Capo Press.

Wilson, W. J. 1987. *The truly disadvantaged: The inner- city, the underclass, and public policy.* Chicago, IL: University of Chicago Press.

Wilson, W. J. 1992. The plight of the inner-city black male. *Proceedings of the American Philosophical Society* 136(3):320–325.

Wilson, W. J. 1996. *When work disappears: The world of the new urban poor.* New York: Knopf.

Young, Jr., A. A. 2004. *The minds of marginalized black men: Making sense of mobility, opportunity, and future life chances.* Princeton, NJ: Princeton University Press.

4

PROMOTING POSITIVE DEVELOPMENT, HEALTH, AND SOCIAL JUSTICE THROUGH DISMANTLING GENETIC DETERMINISM[1]

Richard M. Lerner, PhD

Prominent forums have not adequately countered the egregiously flawed work and counterfactual claims of modern instantiations of genetic determinism, that is, positions that claim that human behavior and development may be reduced to, and explained by, genes. Such formulations are essentialist in character; that is, they hold that there are necessary properties of things and that these properties are logically prior to the existence of the individuals who instantiate them (Lerner, 2016). The essentialist, genetic determinism idea is, then, that the to-be-reduced-to element—the gene—comprises the unit of analysis existing at the fundamental or ultimate level of analysis (i.e., the one that explains human development or, perhaps better, that explains it away or, at the least, that assigns to development a secondary or trivial role in providing a foundation for key features of human structure or function).

An example of such a formulation in developmental science is the idea of evolved probabilistic cognitive mechanisms (EPCMs), which are innate entities said to reside in genes by proponents of evolutionary developmental psychology (EDP) (e.g., Bjorklund, 2015; Bjorklund and Ellis, 2005; Del Giudice and Ellis, 2016). As explained by Witherington and Lickliter (2016), the argument of EDP proponents has been that these EPCMs control the parameters of the higher levels of organization (e.g., cognition or social relationships). The role in human development of these higher levels is only to manage the expression or release of the information contained in the essential, genetic level.

---

1 Preparation of this article was supported in part by grants from the John Templeton Foundation to Richard M. Lerner.

I hope this chapter will be an important, albeit initial, step forward in eliminating genetic determinist ideas from the agenda of contemporary science—and from applications to health and social policies and programs—in America. To establish the basis of such dismantling, I present a view of the role of genes, and of biological processes more generally, within what is, today, the cutting-edge theoretical approach within the study of human development, that is, relational developmental systems theories (Lerner, 2015; Overton, 2015). Throughout the discussion, I contrast this relational developmental systems approach with genetic determinist thinking. I conclude by pointing to the implications of relational developmental systems for enhancing health and social justice for the diverse people of our nation and world.

In my view, social justice focuses on the rights of all groups in a society to have fair access to and a voice in policies governing the distribution of resources essential to their physical and psychological well-being (Fisher and Lerner, 2013). Social justice focuses also on social inequities, characterized as avoidable and unjust social structures and policies that limit access to resources based solely on group or individual characteristics such as race/ethnicity, age, gender, sexual orientation, physical or developmental ability status, and/or immigration status, among others.

SOME PAST AND PRESENT ARGUMENTS OF GENETIC DETERMINISM

Reductionist, genetic determinist ideas have abounded in past and contemporary behavioral and social sciences. These ideas have created inequities in access to individual and social resources and opportunities. As a result, these ideas have created inequities in health, education, and social justice.

For instance, in 1911, the then-renowned scientist Charles Davenport published a rabidly racist book, *Heredity in Relation to Eugenics*, one that included a call for the selective breeding of white people to ensure the health and welfare of the United States through the propagation of people with positive "traits." Davenport's ideas about perfecting humanity by identifying and selectively breeding people who possessed desirable physical and psychological attributes had supporters, but perhaps none so influential as a then-inmate in Landsberg Prison in Germany who wrote a book steeped in the ideas of Davenport: Adolf Hitler published *Mein Kampf* in 1925. In turn, the connection between genetic determinist ideas was furthered in the 1960s, when Nobel Laureate William Shockley of Stanford University argued that intelligence was genetically based and that African Americans had genes that made them less intelligent than white Americans. He discouraged education as a remedy for the low levels of African

American intelligence. Instead, Shockley called for birth control and sterilization (see also Herrnstein and Murray, 1994).

Today, there are few scientists who would make the case for selective breeding of humans or who would recommend ideas popular during Davenport's time, such as forced sterilization or eugenics report cards to focus attention of how well children were doing in manifesting the purportedly positive traits present in their germ line. Nevertheless, there are more recent manifestations of genetic determinist ideas, such as behavioral genetics, heritability analyses of human behavioral attributes, human sociobiology, and evolutionary developmental psychology (see Box 4-1).

BOX 4-1
Examples of Genetic Determinist Ideas in the Study of Human Development

Behavior genetics. A field that seeks to identify the proportion of human behaviors and development that are attributable to genes, to environment, and to the interactions between genes and environment.

Heritability analyses of human behavioral attributes. A method used by behavioral geneticists to identify the percentage of differences between people in a specific sample that are associated with genetic differences between them.

Human sociobiology. A field that seeks to explain human behavior across the lifespan by reference to ideas about how humans evolved.

Evolutionary developmental psychology. A field related to human sociobiology that seeks to explain how evolved genetic mechanisms, inherited at birth, set the range of characteristics that can be developed across the lifespan.

Some of the versions of these ideas come perilously close to making the eugenicist arguments redolent of the Davenport and Shockley eras. One example is Jay Belsky's neo-eugenicist November 2014 op-ed piece in the *New York Times Sunday Review*. Belsky claims that there are some children who have genes that make them unable to gain from social interventions. Consistent with Shockley's rejection of educational interventions for African Americans, Belsky recommends that society should not waste money on attempts to enhance their lives, presumably even when these programs are aimed at reducing inequities in health or education.

Moreover, these genetic determinist ideas find their way into contemporary media. For instance, a 2014 book by journalist Nicholas Wade includes a claim akin to one made by Shockley. Wade (2014) argues that genes shape social behavior, manifested as behavioral traits that are alleged to vary significantly among races. Wade argues that these genes account for racial differences in wealth and economic institutions more generally. In short, if racial groups are either poor or rich, Wade contends that it is because of the evolution of their genes and not social discrimination, racism, lack of education, etc. This book continues to elicit attention despite the erudite and compelling criticism it has received, for instance, in a review of the book by Stanford University geneticist Marcus Feldman (2014).

Feldman's (2014) criticisms do not stand alone. Indeed, the ideas of modern reductionists/genetic determinists such as Belsky and others (e.g., Belsky, 2012; Ellis et al., 2012; Plomin et al., 2012; Rushton, 2000) have been subjected to penetrating criticism by scientists from diverse disciplines (e.g., Bateson, 2015; Ho, 2010; Jablonka and Lamb, 2005; Joseph, 2014; Keller, 2010; Lewontin, 2000; Lickliter and Honeycutt, 2015; Molenaar, 2014; Panofsky, 2014; Woese, 2004).

AN ALTERNATIVE TO GENETIC DETERMINISM: RELATIONAL DEVELOPMENTAL SYSTEMS

Developmental science has three goals. First, developmental scientists seek to *describe* the changes within a person over the course of his or her life. They also seek to describe any differences between people in regard to how they change across life. Second, developmental scientists seek to both *explain* how individuals develop and to *account* for why people differ in their development. For instance, some people show increases, others show decreases, and still others show curvilinear changes in some chapters across life. Why? In addition, what accounts for the differences between people in their pathways across the course of life? Third, developmental science is vitally concerned with applications. Scholars working in this field strive to find ways to promote healthy development for all people. They seek to *optimize* the chances of all people to lead positive and healthy lives (Baltes et al., 1977; Lerner, 2012; Lerner et al., 2014).

At this writing, contemporary developmental science is characterized, theoretically, by the centrality of theories or models derived from the relational developmental systems (RDS) metatheory.[2] The RDS metatheory embraces a new

2   A metatheory is a theory of theories; it is a set of ideas about how theories should be constructed and/or about the ideas that should be included in a theory.

understanding of the role of biology in human development, one predicated on integrative understanding of evolution and of epigenetics, that is, the study of genetic activity caused by processes other than changes in DNA sequence and that result in changes passed on to other generations (Misteli, 2013; see also Jablonka and Lamb, 2005; Meaney, 2010, 2014; Woese, 2004). The link between developmental and biological science enables scholars using RDS-based research to enact applications to optimize human health and development and to promote social justice.

The RDS Metatheory

Because of the contributions of Willis F. Overton (e.g., Overton, 2015; Overton and Müller, 2013) and others (e.g., Gottlieb, 1997, 1998), the sun has set on split, reductionist accounts stressing nature or nurture. The metatheory described by Overton is termed relational developmental systems. Within the RDS metatheory, the integration of different levels of organization frames understanding of life-span human development (Lerner, 2006; Overton, 2015). Figure 4-1 presents an RDS-based model of the fused relations among the levels of organization in the ecology of human development (cf. Bronfenbrenner, 1977, 1979; Gottlieb, 1992; Lerner, 2004; Lerner et al., 2015a).

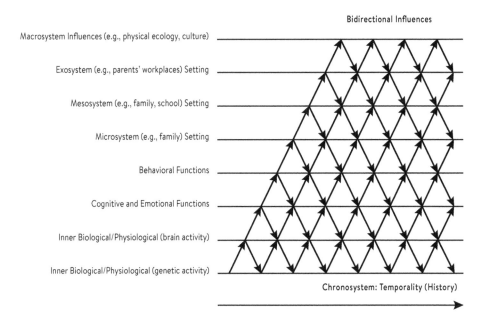

FIGURE 4-1 | A relational developmental systems–based model of the fused relations among the levels of organization in the ecology of human development.
SOURCE: Inspired by Gottlieb (1992), Bronfenbrenner (1977, 1979, 2005), Lerner (2004), and Lerner et al. (2015a).

Accordingly, the conceptual emphasis in RDS-based theories is placed on mutually influential relations between individuals and contexts, represented as individual–context relations. These relations vary across place and across time (Elder et al., 2015); the "arrow of time," or temporality, is history, which is the broadest level within the ecology of human development. History imbues all other levels with change. Such change may be stochastic (e.g., nonnormative life or historical events; Baltes et al., 2006) or systematic, and the potential for systematic change constitutes a potential for (at least relative) plasticity (i.e., the potential for systematic change) across the lifespan. Such plasticity is a strength of human behavior and development (Lerner, 1984, 2012).

Theories derived from an RDS metatheory focus on the "rules"—the processes that govern, or regulate, exchanges between (the functioning of) individuals and their contexts. Brandtstädter (1998) terms these relations "developmental regulations." When developmental regulations involve mutually beneficial individual–context relations, then these developmental regulations are adaptive. Developmental regulations are the fundamental feature of human life; indeed all life exists through bidirectional exchanges with the physical and/or social context (Darwin, 1859; Tobach and Schneirla, 1968). Among humans, these exchanges involve physiological systems and functions (e.g., respiration, circulation, digestion, and reproduction) and behaviors (e.g., social affiliation and cooperation, as might be involved in protection, hunting, and scavenging; Johanson and Edey, 1981), and involve both organismic self-regulation (e.g., hypothalamic functioning, circadian rhythms) and intentional self-regulation (e.g., goal selection, resource recruitment, and executive functioning; Gestsdóttir and Lerner, 2008; McClelland et al., 2015). The developmental course of self-regulation is, in effect, the developmental course of human agency (Sokol et al., 2015).

In short, models derived from RDS metatheory emphasize that all levels of organization within the ecology of human development are systemically integrated across life. As such, any variable from any level is *embodied in*, or fused or integrated with, variables from all other levels; the structure and function of one variable is thus governed, or regulated, by the structure and function of other variables. For the developing person, these developmental regulations mean that individual–context relations are the basic unit of analysis within human development.

As noted, plasticity is always a relative phenomenon within RDS. Temporally ordered events in the life or lives of an individual or a group, respectively, may constrain change as well as provide affordances for it (Lerner, 1984). A system that promotes change can also function to diminish it, a point made as well by Maruyama (1963) in his discussion of deviation amplification and deviation countering processes within systems and, later, by Aldwin (2007) and Aldwin and Gilman (2013) regarding human development systems. However, because of relative plasticity, developmental scientists may be optimistic that instances of individual–context relations may be found or created to promote more positive human development among all people, and to promote social justice by providing opportunities for all individuals to optimize their chances of positive, healthy development (Lerner and Overton, 2008).

The creation of such promotion and optimization efforts rests on the conduct of multidisciplinary research, the use of change-sensitive methodologies, and the translation of research into policies or programs. Contemporary developmental science is marked by such scholarship within and across several substantive areas framing the field. Of particular relevance here is the burgeoning attention to the interrelated areas of evolutionary biology and of epigenetics.

Evolutionary Biology and Epigenetics

Within the integrative RDS metatheory, biological, psychological, and behavioral attributes of the person, in fusion with culture, have a temporal (historical) parameter (Overton, 2015). As such, the fusion among all variables and all levels of organization within the RDS has implications across both ontogeny (the life span of a species) and phylogeny (the evolutionary history of a species) (Ho, 2010; Jablonka and Lamb, 2005). One key implication involves the idea that qualitative changes emerge across the life span through the integration of organism and contextual levels of organization (Lerner, 1984, 2012).

A second key implication is the creation of relative plasticity in phylogeny and ontogeny occurring because of embodied actions (i.e., actions involving the physical body of the individual with his or her social and broader ecological context) resulting in autopoietic (or self-constructing) change in the developmental system (Witherington, 2015). That is, relative plasticity characterizes the relations between organisms and contexts that, across time, create qualitative change in developmental processes within and across generations (Lerner, 1984). This qualitative discontinuity involves what developmental scientists have termed "epigenetic (emergent) change" (e.g., Gottlieb, 1997, 1998; Werner, 1957) in ontogeny. In turn, the action of genetic–context processes that are instances of embodied change within the developmental system is the focus of study in the field of epigenetics (e.g., Meaney, 2010; Misteli, 2013; Slavich and Cole, 2013).

It is important to distinguish the differences in denotation for these two uses of the term "epigenesis." Within the description of developmental change across the life span, the term "epigenesis" refers to the emergence of qualitatively discontinuous characteristics (e.g., developmental stages) across ontogeny (see Gottlieb, 1997, 1998; Lerner, 1984; Lerner and Benson, 2013; Werner, 1957). In turn, Misteli (2013) notes that the term "epi" comes from the Greek and means "over" or "above," and indicates that epigenetic effects are effects that are ones "beyond" the effects of genes. Accordingly, in the literatures of evolutionary biology and of molecular biology, the term "epigenetics" refers to a process involving gene–context relations resulting in the modification of information transmitted by DNA (through messenger RNA, or mRNA) across long, even multigenerational, timescales (e.g., Meaney, 2010, Misteli, 2013; Slavich and Cole, 2013).

Bateson and Gluckman (2011) observe that gene expression is fundamentally shaped by variables external to the cell nucleus (where deoxyribonucleic acid [DNA] is located). They stress, therefore, that "A willingness to move between different levels of analysis has become essential for an understanding of development and evolution" (Bateson and Gluckman, 2011, p. 5). Similarly, Keller (2010) explains that it is erroneous either to conceptualize development as involving separate causal influences or to posit that attributes of the person develop as an outcome of the interaction of causal elements. Indeed, she notes that the concept of interaction is itself flawed, in that its use is predicated on the idea that there exist attributes that are at least conceptually separate. Keller explains that the concept of developmental dynamics precludes such separation. She emphasizes that "From its very beginning, development depends on the complex orchestration of multiple courses of action that involve interactions among many different kinds of elements—including not only preexisting elements (e.g., molecules) but also new elements (e.g., coding sequences) that are formed out of such interactions, temporal sequences of events, dynamical interactions, etc." (Keller, 2010, pp. 6–7).

Moreover, Pigliucci and Müller (2010) note that genes are not as much generators of evolutionary change as they are followers in the evolutionary process. They explain that "evolution progresses through the capture of emergent interactions into genetic-epigenetic circuits, which are passed to and elaborated on in subsequent generations" (Pigliucci and Müller, 2010, p. 14). Similarly, West-Eberhard (2003) connects evolution and the presence of relative plasticity across development. She explains that environmental variables are a major basis of adaptive evolutionary change. As also pointed out by Pigliucci and Müller (2010), West-Eberhard (2003) notes that genetic mutation does not provide either the origin or the evolution of novel adaptive characteristics because "genes are followers not leaders, in evolution" (p. 20). In addition, she explains that the relative plasticity of the phenotype can facilitate evolution by providing immediate changes in the organism (West-Eberhard, 2003). Similarly, Gissis and Jablonka (2011) note that plasticity "is . . . a large topic, but, just as Lamarck anticipated, an understanding of plasticity is now recognized as being fundamental to an understanding of evolution" (p. xiii).

Crystallizing the integration (embodiment) of variables from all levels of organization within the RDS that create epigenetic change across generations, Jablonka and Lamb (2005) present evidence demonstrating that human evolution involves four interrelated dimensions: genes, epigenetics, behavior, and culture. They explain that contemporary research in molecular biology indicates clearly that current, neo-Darwinian assumptions (i.e., ideas about evolution that build on but transcend the specific ideas introduced by Darwin about evolution) about the role of genes in evolution are mistaken. This research demonstrates that cells can transmit information to daughter cells through non-DNA, epigenetic means. Therefore, genetic and epigenetic processes constitute two dimensions of evolution. In addition, animals can transmit information across generations though their behavior, which constitutes a third dimension of evolution. A fourth dimension of evolution is constituted by culture, in that humans "inherit" from their parents symbols and, in particular, language. As such, Jablonka and Lamb (2005) conclude that "It is therefore quite wrong to think about hered-ity and evolution solely in terms of the genetic system. Epigenetic, behavioral, and symbolic inheritance also provide variation on which natural selection can act" (p. 1). Figure 4-1 is again useful in envisioning the relations discussed by Jablonka and Lamb (2005).

These epigenetic effects referred to by Jablonka and Lamb (2005) occur because chemicals in the cell either allow or do not allow DNA to be transcribed into mRNA (Misteli, 2013). For example, acetyl groups (chemicals in the cell that may activate genes), when linked with one of the four base chemicals compos-ing DNA, that is, to cytosine, allow DNA transcription; this process is termed acetylation. In turn, when methyl groups (chemicals in the cells that may silence genes) are linked to cytosine, then there is no transcription of DNA into mRNA. This process is termed methylation. In short, acetylation processes allow DNA to be transcribed into mRNA (and to, therefore, play a role in producing proteins), and methylation processes silence DNA transcription.

If DNA is not transcribed into mRNA, then this DNA cannot play a role in the production of proteins for use by the cell. Because this silencing of gene transcription can persist (can remain stable) across generations (Meaney, 2010; Misteli, 2013; Roth, 2012; Slavich and Cole, 2013), epigenetic influences consti-tute heritable changes explained by processes other than DNA. Indeed, Gissis and Jablonka (2011), in a book discussing the transformations of Lamarckian theory that have arisen in relation to the increasingly more active focus on epigenetic processes in the study of both evolution and development (Meaney, 2010), note that a form of inheritance of acquired characteristics does exist in the form of epigenetic inheritance systems.

This system of epigenetic effects involves chemicals within the cell, within the internal milieu of the body, and within the external ecology within which the body is embedded (Misteli, 2013; Roth, 2012; Slavich and Cole, 2013) or embodied, in the terms used by Overton (2015). For instance, Roth (2012) notes that the genome of infants is modified by epigenetic changes involving experiential and environmental variables. She explains that parental stress, infant separation, or caregiver nurturance or maltreatment can alter methylation patterns that affect neurobiology and behavior across the life span. Similarly, Slavich and Cole (2013) discuss evidence that changes in the expression of hundreds of genes occurs as a function of the physical and social environments inhabited by humans, and they note that "external social conditions, especially our subjective perceptions of these conditions, can influence our most basic internal biological processes—namely, the expression of our genes" (p. 331)—a view that again highlights the implications of embodied biological changes as a focus of actions aimed at enhancing positive human development or social justice.

The evidence concerning epigenetics, embodied action, and plasticity that today is understood as accounting for the features of evolutionary and developmental change necessarily leads to deep skepticism about the "extreme nature" (Rose and Rose, 2000) of the claims of biological determinists, for example, evolutionary psychology (Rose and Rose, 2000), sociobiology (Lerner, 2002; Lerner and von Eye, 1992), and behavior genetics (Molenaar, 2014). Clearly the claims of such reductionists are inconsistent with the now quite voluminous evidence in support of the role of epigenetics in the multiple, integrated dimensions of human evolution, discussed above (Bateson, 2015; Coall et al., 2015; Gissis and Jablonka, 2011; Gunnar et al., 2015; Jablonka and Lamb, 2005; Lickliter and Honeycutt, 2015). Moreover, these claims run counter to research that has importantly begun focusing on the role of the organism's active agency (McClelland et al., 2015), and of culture (Mistry and Dutta, 2015), in creating change within and across generations.

In contrast to the claims of biological reductionists, concepts associated with the RDS metatheory (Overton, 2015) suggest that transmission across generations is accounted for by the plastic embodied processes of the individual functioning in a reciprocal, that is, bidirectional relation with his or her physical and cultural context. Thus, within the RDS perspective, and in the context of contemporary evolutionary scholarship, (e.g., Gissis and Jablonka, 2011; Ho, 2010; Keller, 2010; Lickliter and Honeycutt, 2015; Meaney, 2010, 2014), the "just so" stories (Gould, 1981) of evolutionary psychology are conceptually and empirically flawed. Furthermore, embodiment constitutes the basis for epigenesis within the person's life span (Gottlieb, 1997, 1998), including qualitative discontinuity across ontogeny in relations among biological, psychological, behavioral, and social-cultural variables. Evidence for the relative plasticity of human development within the integrated levels of the ecology of human development makes biologically reductionist accounts (or, equally, completely sociogenic accounts) of parenting, offspring development, or sexuality implausible, at best, and entirely fanciful, at worst (Lerner, 1984, 2006, 2012). This evidence also makes the neo-eugenicist claims of Belsky (2014) scientifically vacuous. Using such claims as a basis for health or social policy is inappropriate at best and irresponsible at worst.

In sum, the RDS metatheory provides an approach to the study of change that capitalizes on the dynamic, mutually influential relations between developing individuals and their complex and changing ecology. As such, this approach to conceptualizing human development may be used to integrate both the agency of individuals (e.g., related to such concepts as grit, executive functioning, soft skills, noncognitive skills, or character) and contextual processes (e.g., involving the social determinants of health) manifested with the designed (i.e., built) and natural ecologies of human development.

The "strands" of theory associated with the RDS metatheory merged in the 1970s, 1980s, and 1990s and created a focus on models emphasizing that time and place matter in regard to shaping the course of life (Bronfenbrenner, 2005; Elder, 1998; Elder and Shanahan, 2006; Elder et al., 2015). A key emphasis in these ideas is that the scientific study of human development may test ideas about the importance of relative plasticity by instantiating evidence-based changes in individual–context relations in attempts to promote positive and healthy development (Lerner et al., 2014).

IMPLICATIONS FOR THE APPLICATION OF RDS-BASED RESEARCH

Among the many split conceptions maintained by viewing the study of development through a reductionist, and essentialist, lens (Overton, 2015) was the split between basic and applied research. However, within models of human development derived from the RDS metatheory, this split joins other ones (e.g., nature–nurture or continuity–discontinuity) in being rejected. When one studies the embodied individual within the developmental system, then explanations of how changes in the individual–context relation (at Time 1) may eventuate in subsequent changes in this relation (at Time 2, Time 3, etc.) are tested by altering the Time 1 person–context relation (again, Figure 4-1 provides an illustration of these temporal, historical relations). When such alterations are conducted in the ecologically valid setting of the individual, these assessments constitute tests of the basic, relational process of human development and, at the same time, applications—interventions—into the course of human development (Lerner and Callina, 2014).

Consider youth development as a sample case (see Lerner et al., 2015b, for a review). Depending on the level of analysis, aggregation, and timescale at which these interventions are implemented, such changes in the ecology of the individual–context relation may involve relationships between individuals (e.g., mentoring relationships), community-based programs (e.g., youth development programs such as 4-H, Boy Scouts, Girl Scouts, YMCA, Girls, Inc., Boys & Girls Clubs, and Big Brothers/Big Sisters), or social policies (e.g., Bronfenbrenner, 2005). There is burgeoning evidence that these initiatives can promote the positive development of diverse young people (e.g., Rhodes and Lowe, 2009; Roth and Brooks-Gunn, 2003; Vandell et al., 2015).

As we have explained, the rationale for applying developmental science to enhance the lives of individuals or groups is predicated on the presence of relative plasticity in human development, a concept that is derived from RDS-based ideas, such as directionally influential individual–context relations and embodiment. The relative plasticity of human development is not only a fundamental strength of human development but also a basis of optimism about human development. Developmental scientists can be hopeful that there are combinations of person and context that can be identified or created (through programs or policies) to enhance the lives of all individuals and groups. In other words, developmental scientists may act to change the course of developmental regulations, of individual–context relations, in manners aimed at optimizing the opportunities for individual and group trajectories across life to reflect health and thriving.

In short, in light of the relative plasticity of human development, neo-eugenicist claims that genes preclude some youth from profiting from health or education programs (e.g., Belsky, 2014) are conceptually inadequate and empirically flawed. There is no constraint imposed by the nature of the human developmental process on the potential productivity of programs or policies aimed at eliminating health and education inequities and thereby furthering social justice. To the contrary, the fundamental plasticity of the individual–context developmental process is a basis for optimism that elimination of such inequities can enhance the health and well-being of diverse youth.

IMPLICATIONS FOR THE PROMOTION OF POSITIVE DEVELOPMENT, HEALTH, AND SOCIAL JUSTICE

Developmental scientists have in the repertoire of models and methods (Molenaar et al., 2014) in their intellectual "tool box" the means to work to promote a better life for all people. When these tools are used within effective collaborations with scholars from other fields, practitioners, policy experts, and community members (Fisher and Lerner, 2013; Fisher et al., 2012; Jensen et al., 1999), developmental scientists may contribute to initiatives that offer to diverse individuals the requisite chances needed to maximize their aspirations for, and to promote their actions aimed at, being active producers of their positive development. Simply, through such collaborations, developmental scientists may act to promote a more socially just world (Lerner, 2002, 2004; Lerner and Overton, 2008).

In this regard, Lerner and Overton (2008) note that theoretically predicated changes in the RDS need to be evaluated in regard to how more positive development may be promoted among individuals whose ecological characteristics (e.g., socioeconomic circumstances or educational opportunities) lower the probability of such development. To contribute significantly to creating a developmental science and to a joint effort involving multiple disciplines, multiple professions, and community collaborations aimed at promoting social justice, scholars need to identify the means to change individual–context relations in manners that enhance the probability that all individuals, no matter their individual characteristics or contextual circumstances (e.g., of poverty, racism, sexism, classism, ageism, and xenophobia) have greater opportunity to experience positive development (e.g., see Fisher et al., 2012).

Developmental science framed by the process-relational RDS paradigm has a clear agenda involving such scholarship. For instance, Fisher et al. (2012) provide a vision for social justice–relevant research in developmental science. Some of the research foci they discuss are

- addressing the pervasive systemic disparities in opportunities for development;
- investigating the origins, structures, and consequences of social inequities in human development;
- identifying societal barriers to health and well-being;
- identifying barriers to fair allocation and access to resources essential to positive development;
- identifying how racist and other prejudicial ideologies and behaviors develop in majority groups;

- studying how racism, heterosexism, classism, and other forms of chronic and acute systemic inequities and political marginalization may have a "weathering" effect on physical and mental health across the life span;
- enacting evidence-based prevention and policy research aimed at demonstrating if systemic oppression can be diminished and psychological and political liberation can be promoted;
- taking a systems-level approach to reducing unjust institutional practices and to promoting individual and collective political empowerment within organizations, communities, and local and national governments;
- evaluating programs and policies that alleviate developmental harms caused by structural injustices; and
- creating and evaluating empirically based interventions that promote a just society that nurtures lifelong healthy development in all of its members.

The epigenetic and embodied developmental changes that characterize individual–context relations within the autopoietic RDS and that provide both a rationale for and optimism about applying developmental science in the service of promoting thriving and social justice for all people require "a theoretical framework more akin to current dynamic-systems models than to traditional conceptions of either behavioral development or evolution" (Harper, 2005, p. 352). Overton (2013) provides this theoretical framework. The RDS metatheory that he has forwarded explains why "the Cartesian-split-mechanistic scientific paradigm that until recently functioned as the standard conceptual framework for subfields of developmental science (including inheritance, evolution, and organismic—prenatal, cognitive, emotional, motivational, sociocultural—development) has been progressively failing as a scientific research program" (Overton, 2013, p. 22). He notes:

An alternative scientific paradigm composed of nested metatheories with relationism at the broadest level and relational developmental systems as a midrange metatheory is offered as a more progressive conceptual framework for developmental science. Termed broadly the "relational developmental systems paradigm," this framework accounts for the findings that are anomalies for the old paradigm; accounts for the emergence of new findings; and points the way to future scientific productivity. (Overton, 2013, p. 22)

CONCLUSIONS

So, where do we go from here? The theoretical orientations and interests of contemporary cohorts of developmental scientists, the aspiration to produce scholarship that matters in the real world, and the needs for evidence-based means to address the challenges of the 21st century have coalesced to make Kurt Lewin's (1952, p. 169) quote, that "There is nothing so practical as a good theory," an oft-proven empirical reality. The scientific and societal value on which developmental science will be judged will be whether its theoretical and methodological tools can, on the one hand, contribute (in collaboration with other disciplines) to effectively dismantling genetic determinist ideas that, at this writing, continue to constrain opportunities for health and positive development among diverse individuals and, as well, to denigrate, disempower, and deny hope to them.

On the other hand, developmental science will also be judged by the scholarship it leaves in the place of genetic determinism. This science must accurately reflect the diversity and dynamism of human development, must build bridges across disciplines, professions, and with diverse communities to ensure integrative, multidisciplinary, collaborative approaches to promoting human health and social justice (Fisher and Lerner, 2013; Fisher et al., 2012), and be centered on promoting thriving across the life span for all people. Therefore, promoting human thriving and health and social justice is, and will be, the most significant lens through which the contributions of developmental science, and of the broad collaboration of which it must be a part, will be viewed.

REFERENCES

Aldwin, C. M. 2007. *Stress, coping, and development: An integrative approach*, 2nd ed. New York: Guilford.

Aldwin, C. M., and D. F. Gilmer. 2013. *Health, illness, and optimal aging: Biological and psychosocial perspectives*, 2nd ed. New York: Springer.

Baltes, P. B., H. W. Reese, and J. R. Nesselroade. 1977. *Life-span developmental psychology: Introduction to research methods*. Monterey, CA: Brooks/Cole.

Baltes, P. B., U. Lindenberger, and U. M. Staudinger. 2006. Life span theory in developmental psychology. In *Handbook of child psychology, Vol. 1: Theoretical models of human development*, 6th ed., edited by W. Damon and R. M. Lerner. Hoboken, NJ: John Wiley & Sons. Pp. 569–664.

Bateson, P. 2015. Ethology and human development. In *Handbook of child psychology and developmental science, Vol. 1: Theory and method*, 7th ed., edited by W. F. Overton and P. C. Molenaar. Hoboken, NJ: John Wiley & Sons. Pp. 208–243.

Bateson, P., and P. Gluckman. 2011. *Plasticity, development and evolution*. Cambridge, UK: Cambridge University Press.

Belsky, J. 2012. The development of human reproductive strategies: Progress and prospects. *Current Directions in Psychological Science* 21(5):310–316.

Belsky, J. 2014. The downside of resilience. *New York Times Sunday Review*, November 30.

Bjorklund, D. F. 2015. Developing adaptations. *Developmental Review* 38:13–35.

Bjorklund, D. F., and B. J. Ellis. 2005. Evolutionary psychology and child development: An emerging synthesis. In *Origins of the social mind: Evolutionary psychology and child development*, edited by B. J. Ellis and D. F. Bjorklund. New York: Guilford Press. Pp. 3–18.

Brandtstädter, J. 1998. Action perspectives on human development. In *Handbook of child psychology, Vol. 1: Theoretical models of human development*, 6th ed., edited by W. Damon and Richard M. Lerner. New York: John Wiley & Sons. Pp. 807–863.

Bronfenbrenner, U. 1977. Toward an experimental ecology of human development. *American Psychologist* 32:513–531.

Bronfenbrenner, U. 1979. *The ecology of human development: Experiments by nature and design.* Cambridge, MA: Harvard University Press.

Bronfenbrenner, U., ed. 2005. *Making human beings human.* Thousand Oaks, CA: Sage Publications.

Coall, D. A., A. C. Callan, T. E. Dickins, and J. S. Chisholm. 2015. Evolution and prenatal development: An evolutionary perspective. In *Handbook of child psychology and developmental science, Vol. 3: Socioemotional Processes,* 7th ed., edited by R. M. Lerner and M. E. Lamb. Hoboken, NJ: John Wiley & Sons. Pp. 57–105.

Darwin, C. 1859. *The origin of species by means of natural selection or the preservation of favoured races in the struggle for life.* London: J. Murray.

Del Giudice, M., and B. J. Ellis. 2016. Evolutionary foundations of developmental psychopathology. In *Developmental psychopathology, Vol. 12: Developmental neuroscience,* 3rd ed. New York: John Wiley & Sons. Pp. 1–58.

Elder, G. H. Jr. 1998. The life course and human development. In *Handbook of child psychology, Vol. 1.: Theoretical models of human development,* 5th ed., edited by W. Damon and R. M. Lerner, New York: John Wiley & Sons. Pp. 939–991.

Elder, G. H. Jr., and M. J. Shanahan. 2006. The life course and human development. In *Handbook of child psychology, Vol. 1: Theoretical models of human development,* 6th ed., edited by W. Damon and R. M. Lerner. Hoboken, NJ: John Wiley & Sons. Pp. 665–715.

Elder, G. H., M. J. Shanahan, and J. A. Jennings. 2015. Human development in time and place. In *Handbook of child psychology and developmental science, Vol. 4: Ecological settings and processes in developmental systems,* 7th ed., edited by M. H. Bornstein and T. Leventhal. Hoboken, NJ: John Wiley & Sons. Pp. 6–54.

Ellis, B. J., G. L. Schlomer, E. H. Tilley, and E.A. Butler. 2012. Impact of fathers on risky sexual behavior in daughters: A genetically and environmentally controlled sibling study. *Development and Psychopathology* 24:317–332.

Feldman, M. 2014. Echoes of the past: Hereditarianism and a troublesome inheritance. *PLoS Genetics* 10:e1004817.

Fisher, C. B., and R. M. Lerner. 2013. Promoting positive development through social justice: An introduction to a new ongoing section of *Applied Developmental Science.* *Applied Developmental Science* 17(2):57–59.

Fisher, C. B., N. A. Busch, J. L. Brown, and D. S. Jopp. 2012. Applied developmental science: Contributions and challenges for the 21st century. In *Handbook of psychology, Vol. 6: Developmental psychology,* 2nd ed., edited by I. B. Weiner. New York: John Wiley & Sons. Pp. 516–546.

Gestsdóttir, G., and R. M. Lerner. 2008. Positive development in adolescence: The development and role of intentional self-regulation. *Human Development* 51:202–224.

Gissis, S. B., and E. Jablonka. 2011. Preface. In *Transformations of Lamarckism: From subtle fluids to molecular biology*, edited by S. B. Gissis and E. Jablonka. Cambridge, MA: MIT Press. Pp. xi-xiv.

Gottlieb, G. 1992. *Individual development and evolution: The genesis of novel behavior*. New York: Oxford University Press.

Gottlieb, G. 1997. *Synthesizing nature-nurture: Prenatal roots of instinctive behavior*. Mahwah, NJ: Lawrence Erlbaum Associates.

Gottlieb, G. 1998. Normally occurring environmental and behavioral influences on gene activity: From central dogma to probabilistic epigenesis. *Psychological Review* 105:792–802.

Gould, S. J. 1981. *The mismeasure of man*. New York: Norton.

Gunnar, M. R., J. R. Doom, and E. A. Esposito. 2015. Psychoneuroendocrinology of stress: Normative development and individual differences. In *Handbook of child psychology and developmental science, Vol. 3: Socioemotional processes*, 7th ed., edited by M. E. Lamb. Hoboken, NJ: John Wiley & Sons. Pp. 106–151.

Harper, L. V. 2005. Epigenetic inheritance and the intergenerational transfer of experience. *Psychological Bulletin* 131:340–360.

Herrnstein, R. J., and C. Murray. 1994. *The bell curve: Intelligence and class structure in American life*. New York: Free Press.

Ho, M. W. 2010. Development and evolution revisited. In *Handbook of developmental systems, behavior and genetics*, edited by K. E. Hood, C. T. Halpern, G. Greenberg, and R. M. Lerner. Malden, MA: Wiley-Blackwell. Pp. 61–109.

Jablonka, E., and M. J. Lamb. 2005. *Evolution in four dimensions: Genetic, epigenetic, behavioral, and symbolic variation in the history of life*. Cambridge, MA: MIT Press.

Jensen, P., K. Hoagwood, and E. Trickett. 1999. Ivory towers or earthen trenches? Community collaborations to foster "real world" research. *Applied Developmental Science* 3(4):206–212.

Johanson, D. C., and M. A. Edey. 1981. *Lucy: The beginnings of humankind*. New York: Simon & Schuster.

Joseph, J. 2014. *The trouble with twin studies: A reassessment of twin research in the social and behavioral sciences*. New York: Routledge.

Keller, E. F. 2010. *The mirage of a space between nature and nurture*. Durham, NC: Duke University Press.

Lerner, R. M. 1984. *On the nature of human plasticity*. New York: Cambridge University Press.

Lerner, R. M. 2002. *Concepts and theories of human development*, 3rd ed. Mahwah, NJ: Lawrence Erlbaum Associates.

Lerner, R. M. 2004. *Liberty: Thriving and civic engagement among America's youth*. Thousand Oaks, CA: Sage Publications.

Lerner, R. M. 2006. Developmental science, developmental systems, and contemporary theories of human development. In *Handbook of child psychology, Vol. 1: Theoretical models of human development*, 6th ed., edited by W. Damon and R. M. Lerner. Hoboken, NJ: John Wiley & Sons. Pp. 1–17.

Lerner, R. M. 2012. Essay review: Developmental science: Past, present, and future. *International Journal of Developmental Science* 6(1–2):29–36.

Lerner, R. M. 2015. Promoting social justice by rejecting genetic reductionism: A challenge for developmental science. *Human Development* 58:67–69.

Lerner, R. M. 2016. Complexity embraced and complexity reduced: A tale of two approaches to human development. A commentary on Witherington and Lickliter. *Human Development* 59:242–249.

Lerner, R. M., and J. B. Benson. 2013. Introduction: Embodiment and epigenesis: A view of the issues. In *Advances in child development and behavior, Vol. 44: Embodiment and epigenesis: Theoretical and methodological issues in understanding the role of biology within the relational developmental system*, edited by R. M. Lerner and J. B. Benson. London, UK: Elsevier. Pp. 1–20.

Lerner, R. M., and Callina, K. S. 2014. The study of character development: Towards tests of a relational developmental systems model. *Human Development* 57(6):322–346.

Lerner, R. M., and W. F. Overton. 2008. Exemplifying the integrations of the relational developmental system: Synthesizing theory, research, and application to promote positive development and social justice. *Journal of Adolescent Research* 23(3):245–255.

Lerner, R. M., and A. von Eye. 1992. Sociobiology and human development: Arguments and evidence. *Human Development* 35:12–33.

Lerner, R. M., J. P. Agans, L. M. DeSouza, and R. M. Hershberg. 2014. Developmental science in 2025: A predictive review. *Research in Human Development* 11:255–272.

Lerner, R. M., S. K. Johnson, and M. H. Buckingham. 2015a. Relational developmental systems-based theories and the study of children and families: Lerner and Spanier (1978) revisited. *Journal of Family Theory and Review* 7:83–104.

Lerner, R. M., J. V. Lerner, E. Bowers, and G. J. Geldhof. 2015b. Positive youth development and relational developmental systems. In *Handbook of child psychology and developmental science, Vol. 1: Theory and method*, 7th ed., edited by W. F. Overton and P. C. Molenaar. Hoboken, NJ: John Wiley & Sons. Pp. 607–651.

Lewin, K. 1952. *Field theory in social science: Selected theoretical papers*. London: Tavistock.

Lewontin, R. C. 2000. *The triple helix*. Cambridge, MA: Harvard University Press.

Lickliter, R., and H. Honeycutt. 2015. Biology, development, and human systems. In *Handbook of child psychology and developmental science, Vol. 1: Theory and method*, 7th ed., edited by W. F. Overton and P. C. Molenaar. Hoboken, NJ: John Wiley & Sons. Pp. 162–207.

Maruyama, M. 1963. The second cybernetics: Deviation-amplifying mutual causal processes. *American Scientist* 5(2):164–179.

McClelland, M. M., G. J. Geldhof, C. E. Cameron, and S. B. Wanless. 2015. Development and self-regulation. In *Handbook of child psychology and developmental science, Vol. 1: Theory and method*, 7th ed., edited by W. F. Overton and P. C. Molenaar. Hoboken, NJ: John Wiley & Sons. Pp. 523–565.

Meaney, M. 2010. Epigenetics and the biological definition of gene × environment interactions. *Child Development* 81(1):41–79.

Meaney, M. 2014. Epigenetics offer hope for disadvantaged children. Children and Family Blog, October 10. Available from http://childandfamilyblog.com/epigenetics-offer-hope-disadvantaged-children.

Misteli, T. 2013. The cell biology of genomes: Bringing the double helix to life. *Cell* 152:1209–1212.

Mistry, J., and R. Dutta. 2015. Human development and culture. In *Handbook of child psychology and developmental science, Vol. 1: Theory and method*, 7th ed., edited by W. F. Overton and P. C. Molenaar. Hoboken, NJ: John Wiley & Sons. Pp. 369–406.

Molenaar, P. C. M. 2014. Dynamic models of biological pattern formation have surprising implications for understanding the epigenetics of development. *Research in Human Development* 11(1):50–62.

Molenaar, P. C. M., K. Newell, and R. M. Lerner, eds. 2014. *Handbook of developmental systems theory and methodology*. New York: Guilford Press.

Overton, W. F. 2013. A new paradigm for developmental science: Relationism and relational-developmental-systems. *Applied Developmental Science* 17(2):94–107.

Overton, W. F. 2015. Process and relational developmental systems. In *Handbook of child psychology and developmental science, Vol. 1: Theory and method*, 7th ed., edited by W. F. Overton and P. C. Molenaar. Hoboken, NJ: John Wiley & Sons. Pp. 9–62.

Overton, W. F., and U. Müller. 2013. Development across the life span: Philosophy, concepts, theory. In *Handbook of psychology, Vol. 6: Developmental psychology,* edited by R. M. Lerner, M. A. Easterbrooks, and J. Mistry. New York: John Wiley & Sons. Pp. 19–58.

Panofsky, A. 2014. *Misbehaving science: Controversy and the development of behavior genetics.* Chicago, IL: University of Chicago Press.

Pigliucci, M., and Müller, G. B. 2010. Elements of an extended evolutionary synthesis. In *Evolution—The extended synthesis,* edited by M. Pigliucci and G. B. Müller. Cambridge, MA: MIT Press. Pp. 3–17.

Plomin, R., J. C. DeFries, V. S. Knopik, and J. M. Neiderhiser. 2012. *Behavioral genetics,* 6th ed. New York: Worth.

Rhodes, J. E., and S. R. Lowe. 2009. Mentoring in adolescence. In *Handbook of adolescent psychology, Vol. 2: Contextual influences on adolescent development,* 3rd ed., edited by R. M. Lerner and L. Steinberg. Hoboken, NJ: John Wiley & Sons. Pp. 152–190.

Rose, H., and S. Rose. 2000. Introduction. In *Alas poor Darwin: Arguments against evolutionary psychology,* edited by H. Rose and S. Rose. London: Vintage. Pp. 1–13.

Roth, J. L., and J. Brooks-Gunn. 2003. What exactly is a youth development program? Answers from research and practice. *Applied Developmental Science* 7:94–111.

Roth, T. L. 2012. Epigenetics of neurobiology and behavior during development and adulthood. *Developmental Psychobiology* 54:590–597.

Rushton, J. P. 2000. *Race, evolution, and behavior,* 2nd special abridged ed. New Brunswick, NJ: Transaction Publishers.

Slavich, G. M., and S. W. Cole. 2013. The emerging field of human social genomics. *Clinical Psychological Science* 1:331–348.

Sokol, B. W., S. Hammond, J. Kuebli, and L. Sweetman, 2015. The development of agency. In *Handbook of child psychology and developmental science, Vol. 1: Theory and method*, 7th ed., edited by W. F. Overton and P. C. Molenaar. Hoboken, NJ: John Wiley & Sons. Pp. 284–322.

Tobach, E., and T. C. Schneirla. 1968. The biopsychology of social behavior of animals. In *Biologic basis of pediatric practice,* edited by R. E. Cooke and S. Levin. New York: McGraw-Hill. Pp. 68–82.

Vandell, D. L., R. W. Larson, J. L. Mahoney, and T. R. Watts. 2015. Children's activities. In *Handbook of child psychology and developmental science,* Vol. 4: *Ecological settings and processes in developmental systems,* 7th ed., edited by M. H. Bornstein and T. Leventhal. Hoboken, NJ: John Wiley & Sons. Pp. 305–344.

Wade, N. 2014. *A troublesome inheritance: Genes, race and human history.* New York: Penguin Books.

Werner, H. 1957. The concept of development from a comparative and organismic point of view. In *The concept of development,* edited by D. B. Harris. Minneapolis: University of Minnesota. Pp. 125–148.

West-Eberhard, M. J. 2003. *Developmental plasticity and evolution.* New York: Oxford University Press.

Witherington, D. C. 2015. Dynamic systems in developmental science. In *Handbook of child psychology and developmental science, Vol. 1: Theory and method,* 7th ed., edited by W. F. Overton and P. C. Molenaar. Hoboken, NJ: John Wiley & Sons. Pp. 63–112.

Witherington, D. C., and R. Lickliter. 2016. Integrating development and evolution in psychological science: Evolutionary developmental psychology, developmental systems, and explanatory pluralism. *Human Development* 59:200–234.

Woese, C. R. 2004. A new biology for a new century. *Microbiology and Molecular Biology Reviews* 68(2):173–186.

5

PHILOSOPHICAL PERSPECTIVES ON SOCIAL JUSTICE: A FRAMEWORK FOR DISCUSSING A CHILDREN, YOUTH, AND FAMILIES HEALTH POLICY AND RESEARCH AGENDA

Robert Seidel, MLA, Patrick H. Tolan, PhD, Angela Diaz, MD, PhD, MPH, and Velma McBride Murry, PhD

Discussions of health policy often invoke sentiments of "social justice" and "equity" as primary principles or long-term goals. Implicit in such discussions is an underlying assumption that there is consensus on what a just society might look like and what achieving justice or equity would mean in regard to health opportunities and outcomes. An accompanying presumption, at least implied, is that a body of principles of social justice on which we agree also exists. Yet, outside of academic political philosophy lectures and journals, the articulation of such principles is rare. Even rarer is the explicit connection of these principles to policy, research, and practice decisions. We contend not only that Americans disagree about what is just and equitable on these issues but also that there is a need to engage in careful consideration of what we mean by health equity in research, practice, promotion, and policy. In this endeavor, greater consideration is needed to clarify how these terms and their components are defined and actuated across varying constructions of social equity and justice. Even without consensus on a definition of social justice, discussions of its role in health can only benefit from some common awareness of the major interpretations. This essay provides a brief overview of some major schools of philosophical thought about social justice and equity to emphasize that there is a wide range of perspectives. These perspectives hold different ideas regarding the implications of social justice for health policy, research, and practice. While each school of thought has different definitions of social justice, there are shared concerns about how we ought to live together and what is fair, and that the manner in which resources and responsibilities are distributed and accessed can differ substantially.

While we acknowledge that our framework is an oversimplification of very complex issues, we begin the dialogue on the role of political philosophies regarding social justice and equity by selecting perspectives across different eras and cultures that fall into two broad varieties: those (generally with fullest expression in the European Enlightenment) that emphasize the rights and well-being of the individual, which we term *individual-centric*, and those that emphasize the well-being of the community or society, which we term *community-centric*.

Not surprisingly, there have been many thoughtful and sophisticated efforts to identify the right balance of these two perspectives or to reconcile them. However, for the present consideration, we focus on the contrast of basic values as a framework for organizing our discussion. Our intent is to increase our understanding of ways multiple political philosophies implicitly or explicitly offer different definitions of health equity and thereby imply different strategies and approaches to address social justice in health. That we are providing a brief summary suggests that there are inevitably omissions of details and nuances. Notwithstanding, the intent is less to provide a comprehensive or authoritative rendering of fine distinctions than to bring out the range of political perspectives and values that lead to different connotations of "social justice." These variations in assumptions and values are rarely considered in discussions of health equity research and related practice and policy. This void served as the impetus for our essay, and our goal is to bring that consideration back into overt deliberation.

INDIVIDUAL-CENTRIC PHILOSOPHIES

U.S. society is marked by what is termed in political philosophy as liberalism, or a central concern for the protection and enhancement of the freedom of its citizens as individuals. This is not "liberalism" as it is commonly connoted in the current political debates in our country. As a philosophical term, "liberalism" embraces what most Americans consider to be both conservative and liberal policies and values. Further, philosophical notions of liberalism can consider government as both a potential threat to and protector of individual freedoms. This broad category embraces a number of more-specific perspectives, including libertarianism, John Rawls's idea of justice as fairness (Rawls, 1971), and the capabilities approach championed by Amartya Sen (Sen, 2009) and Martha Nussbaum (Nussbaum, 2007).

Traditional American Liberalism

Within the overall liberalism that encompasses and frames most policy debates in our country, there is the more commonly identified form of liberalism that focuses on fully realizing the promises in the Constitution, Bill of Rights, and other documents for all members of society. This can be seen as the philosophy motivating movements such as the Civil Rights Movement; Women's Rights Movement; and Lesbian, Gay, Bisexual, Transgender, and Queer Rights Movement, as well as those putting religious freedom in contention with other rights and freedoms. What binds these efforts is the view or recognition of the discrepancies between the principles, laws, and policies of the United States in regard to individual freedom (and therefore equal justice) and equal access to those freedoms. The modern rights movements recognize the conflict between individual freedom and the actual treatment of groups of people based on race, gender, sexuality, age, religion, and other natural or socially constructed characteristics.

In regard to health discrepancies, modern liberalism views inequities in opportunity for healthy development as impediments to freedoms of some segments of society enjoyed by others (Sen, 2009). Governmental actions to improve health opportunities and health care access for those who are disadvantaged would, from this perspective, be seen as a necessary action to ensure this freedom is equitably enjoyed by all (Braverman, 2006).

Libertarianism

The libertarian perspective is often contrasted with traditional liberalism. The various strands of modern libertarianism, including Ayn Rand's objectivism (Rand, 1961), emphasize individual choice over equal opportunity or access as the hallmark of guaranteed freedom (Daniels, 1985). While there are variations within this branch of liberalism as to how absolute that emphasis is in regard to health, the emphasis is on individuals' right to control their bodies as well as their resources/capital, as long as their actions do not interfere with other individuals' same rights. Within a broader opposition to government involvement, taxation-based financing, compulsory activities, and regulations that curtail choice, the libertarian approach to health care equity as a social-justice issue is to promote choice and focus any governmental or legal involvement to ensuring fair rules for commerce (Buchanan, 1984). This approach values the freedom of choice over potential inequities that may be sustained due to differences in status or capability but also argues that individual choice in a free-commerce market will lead to greater equity and justice.

Because libertarianism casts health influences, health care access, and health opportunities over the life span as understandable as commerce between individuals and that maximal individual freedom is the most essential value (and best solution), health equity solutions from this perspective tend to be in the form of allowing many choices, minimizing requirements for health care, insurance, features of such insurance, or provision of health care to all. While there is recognition of historical and political bases for inequities of health opportunities, access, and outcomes, this general framework is still offered as the most appropriate and promising approach to health equity and social justice (Daniels, 1985).

Modern Liberalism

Justice as Fairness

Late-20th-century academic political philosophy, particularly in the United States, has been significantly influenced by John Rawls. Rawls sought to temper liberalism's focus on individual rights with a consideration of fairness. To show the importance of fairness, he utilized a thought experiment (Rawls, 1971). In this experiment, he posed the question: *If a group of people were behind a veil of ignorance, knowing nothing about their own specific characteristics (age, gender, race, wealth, ability, religion, likes and dislikes, plans for the future, and so on), what kind of social contract would they adopt before their actual characteristics were revealed?* Not knowing, for example, whether one is rich or poor, deaf or hearing, one might want to both protect oneself by setting rules to minimize vulnerability as well as maximize opportunity along a variety of dimensions.

Based on this thought, Rawls came to the conclusion that two general principles would emerge from deliberations behind the veil of ignorance. The first is that "Each person is to have an equal right to the most extensive basic liberty compatible with a similar liberty for others" (Rawls, 1971, p. 302). The second principle, which he refers to as the "difference principle," is that social and economic inequalities are to be arranged so that they are to be of the greatest benefit to the least-advantaged members of society. Also, offices and positions must be open to everyone under conditions of fair equality of opportunity. Thus, in Rawls' analysis, there is a balance of individual liberties with equality of opportunity, with particular attention to reducing inequities.

From this critical view, rewards should be provided to the extent they reduce inequities or benefit the least advantaged. Doctors should receive greater income than many other people, if and only if that is what it takes to provide adequate health care for the least advantaged. Furthermore, one should not be able to buy one's way into better health care or to advantageous social positions that create privilege over others. From Rawls's perspective, health equity would reside in policies and practices that accorded the most disadvantaged access to opportunities for healthy development, health care and awareness, and quality of life and longevity that align with the most privileged in society (Braverman, 2006). To advance this school of thought, research is needed to identify factors and processes that would enable and improve the circumstances of the disadvantaged and evaluate practice and policies to determine the extent to which they are designed to do so.

The Capabilities Approach

Martha Nussbaum, a senior member of the philosophy faculty at the University of Chicago, and Nobel Prize–winning economist Amartya Sen developed and use the capabilities approach "to provide the philosophical underpinning for an account of core human entitlements that should be respected and implemented by the governments of all nations, as a bare minimum of what respect for human dignity requires" (2007, p. 70). Rather than using the conventional liberal language of human rights, Nussbaum promotes "an approach that focuses on *human capabilities*, that is, what people are actually able to do and to be, in a way informed by an intuitive idea of a life that is worthy of the dignity of the human being" (2007, p. 70). Nussbaum explicitly places the central human capabilities as "the source of political principles for a liberal pluralistic society" (2007, p. 70). She notes that a list of central capabilities will always be a work in progress, but offered this one in 2007:

1. Life (ability to live a life of normal length)
2. Bodily Health (ability to have good health with adequate nourishment and shelter)
3. Bodily Integrity (ability to move freely from place to place, be secure from violent assault, and have opportunities for sexual satisfaction and reproductive choice)
4. Senses, Imagination, and Thought (ability to use the senses, imagine, think, and reason in a way cultivated by adequate education to be creative in context of freedom of expression; ability to enjoy pleasure and avoid nonbeneficial pain)
5. Emotions (ability to love, grieve, experience longing, gratitude, and justified anger; having emotional development not blighted by fear and anxiety)
6. Practical Reason (ability to form a conception of the good and to plan one's own life)
7. Affiliation (ability to engage in various forms of social interaction and feel empathy; ability to freely assemble and engage politically with others; having the social bases of self-respect and nonhumiliation, which entails

nondiscrimination on bases of gender, race, sexual orientation, ethnicity, age, religion, and so on)

8. Other Species (ability to live with concern for animals, plants, and the environment)
9. Play (ability to laugh, play, and enjoy recreation)
10. Control over One's Environment (political: ability to participate effectively in political decisions that govern one's life; ability to hold property on an equal basis with others; ability to seek employment on an equal basis with others and work as a human being, using practical reason and in meaningful relationships with others)

The capabilities approach posits that social justice entails society offering all individuals the opportunity to develop, utilize, and put into effect these essential capabilities, regardless of happenstance of birth, including social standing or inherent abilities. This means that equity implies differential opportunity as needed to compensate for or minimize advantages and disadvantages of persons and stations. An important ethical implication of that society is that it must be embraced by a majority, if not all, and is one that advances equity in status or outcome. Like Rawls, proponents of the capabilities approach embrace fairness as a countervailing or additional consideration along with individual liberty in determining justice and equity.

Jennifer Prah Ruger has undertaken application of the capabilities approach to health and health care. In her 2010 book *Health and Social Justice*, she wrote of "the need for all individuals . . . to understand the obligations each of us has to help realize the right to health for every individual in every society in the global community" (Ruger, 2010, p. 122).

Ruger's statements constitute a philosophy that comes closest to that expressed in the definition offered by Braverman (2006), which defined health equity as a basic human right with the benchmark being the quality of health opportunity, care, and well-being enjoyed by the more privileged but with particular interest in the needs of the disadvantaged.

These two poles—libertarianism and modern liberalism—approach the promotion of freedom quite differently and, in turn, have different implications for what constitutes social justice and how health equity should be viewed. Such implications lean toward one side or the other in primary orientation but include compromising views or mixed principles. These variants include *how* much fairness is located in individual choice versus individual, equal-opportunity access and how regulation of commerce and personal behavior affects equality and justice in health opportunities, access to care, and outcomes.

COMMUNITY-CENTRIC PHILOSOPHIES

Most cultures in the history of humanity have been community-centric in some sense, rather than individual-centric. Some of these are small-scale tribal hunting and gathering societies, Buddhist and Confucian cultures, and socialist and communist state societies. Yet, across these community-centric societies, differences in social organization and the role of government vary enormously. These philosophies each put primary value on the flourishing of the community rather than starting with and giving primacy to the individual. Within this, there is variation, though, in how individual and collective endeavors are seen as contributing to the full realization of human potential.

Tribal Social Organization

Societies with a relatively low level of technology and, hence, productivity of labor, whether they are limited to hunting and gathering or utilize primitive horticulture among their means of subsistence, require all able-bodied individuals to cooperate in producing what they need as a community to survive. Having no surplus production, such societies cannot engage in commodity exchange. Individual choice or liberty is not considered essential or even relevant. An example barely surviving today is the Bambuti people of the tropical rainforest in the Congo (Mukenge, 2002; Turnbull, 1961), who live in bands of a few dozen people. The Bambuti are an egalitarian society in which the band is the highest form of social organization. Men and women basically have equal power. Issues are discussed, and decisions are made by consensus at fire camps; men and women engage in the conversations equivalently. If there is a disagreement or offense, then the offender or uncooperative member may be banished, beaten, or scorned (Mukenge, 2002).

While such organization and its implied political philosophy may seem irrelevant to American society and the issue of health equity, the pure egalitarianism and paramount interdependency are useful to highlight. A major issue within health equity–definition discussions and in policies related to health care is shared interdependency—how much health of the other is each person's concern and how health standing and health costs to the society are affected by recognizing that interdependency.

Confucianism

Confucianism, with its roots in Chinese feudal culture several centuries BCE, continues to have influence even after the remarkable political and economic revolutions in China during the last century (Rosemont, 1991). A central concept is that if people behave morally in their personal lives, then the life of the nation would be orderly and peaceful. The political order rests on the moral conduct of individuals that translates to societal moral order. A central Confucian concept is what is known in Western society as *The Golden Rule*: "Never impose on others what you would not choose for yourself."

For Confucians, this rule is the foundation of a harmonious and, therefore, healthy society. The objective was to enable a harmonious, healthy society, not simply the personal ethic of treating others as you would like to be treated. Under the feudal society in which Confucian philosophy formed and became influential, a harmonious society meant that everyone should know their place in the hierarchy and organization based on ancestry, gender, land ownership, and other status considerations. Thus, it was less about equity than about working in one's assigned role and place to maintain the order.

In addition to concern for social and political harmony, a key concept that places Confucianism as a community-centric philosophy is its understanding of personal identity. In contrast to individual-centric, rights-oriented concepts of justice and equity, Confucianism defines persons as the sum of their relationships and roles in family, community, and society (Rosemont, 1991). A person is defined, first of all, as the child of their parents, then as the sibling of their brothers and/or sisters, then by who they have as friends, neighbors, which teacher they are the student of, who they are the colleague of, the boss they are the underling of, and through numerous other relationships. Identity does not emanate from personality or individual choice and proclivities, but is intimately tied to and the sum of one's relationships in the family and community.

Applied to health equity, what is of interest here is what promotes and maintains order in society. Healthy development opportunities, health education and care, and differences in health status, risks, and outcome are all judged by how these may affect the overall success and capability of the group or society. Individual status is of importance only in how it enables or impedes that overall status. Perhaps most relevant to the health equity discussion in this country is the justification of less concern for particular individuals based on an implicit assumption that inequity may not translate to harm overall, whereas from an individual-oriented perspective, this would be seen as inhumane or discriminatory.

Buddhism

Buddhism is another philosophical perspective that may be informative for addressing social justice and health equity. Within Buddhism, many branches and sub-branches of philosophy have sprouted, emphasizing different traditions.

Some focus on the importance of individuals' ethical life choices, while others stress communal well-being. Across Buddhism there are threads connecting the well-being of the global community to the individual's decisions and actions. An example of this kind of thought in Buddhist tradition is an apocryphal story of a monarch who provided no help for the poor (Ling, 1993). So, poverty was widespread. A poor man was arrested for theft and brought before the king. The man told his story of need, and the king gave him money. So, more and more poor people committed theft in order to receive money from the king. To abate this, the king ordered his men to cut off the heads of thieves. Thieves then armed themselves to fight the king's men. So, from indifference to the poor grew theft, murder, runaway violence, and the shortening of life spans. The story goes on, introducing a host of other social evils, all spawned from indifference to the poor. The lesson, of course, is that society must, for its overall well-being, care for the poor.

This notion that there is interconnection among all people, that circumstances of one affect and are the concern of the others brings a humanitarian orientation to conversations about health and well-being. More specifically, Buddhism emphasizes how incorrect perceptions of others underlie hatred, violence, and unconcern (Hanh, 2006). This is an understanding of health equity that extends beyond equal rights or individual opportunity to view one's health and well-being as not separable from any other person's. From this approach, taking care of other people's health is, at the same time, taking care of our own health. This philosophy can be seen as influential, if not overt, in many models of health equity.

Utilitarianism

Utilitarianism is a community-centric European philosophy. Popularly known as the philosophy of "the greatest good for the greatest number," the idea is that what is desirable in specific situations and the world in general is whatever maximizes pleasure and minimizes pain (Sandel, 2009). While having appeal in providing a simple maxim, utilitarianism faces three challenges in its application. First, there is the question of defining "the good." What is considered pleasurable or desirable by some may not be by others. And, of course, there is the question of by whom and how that judgment is rendered. A subset of this school of thought argues that one can discriminate between higher and lower pleasures. However, as applied to health equity, the challenge remains that, of multiple potentially desirous results, utilitarianism offers little guidance on what is good.

The second challenge of utilitarianism is measurement. If we are to maximize utility in society or even a local community, we must have a way to measure and compare utility among individuals. While some things that affect utility are commensurable, e.g., the number of calories a person has access to daily, others clearly are not. A person has a unique array of needs and preferences. Groups of people also vary in their definition of utility, e.g., in types of cuisine or art. So, if we are to use scarce societal resources to maximize overall utility, how do we assign relative values? How value is assigned has implications for equity, of course, but also determines the degree to which equity will be realized (measured as achieved). Utilitarianism leaves this dependent on how one defines good.

The third major issue, one which has perhaps kept utilitarianism from being embraced at a societal level, is the question of means. A classic case is that of the sailors adrift in a lifeboat. As their rations ran low, they considered turning to cannibalism, so that at least some of them might survive longer with the hope of rescue. Classic utilitarianism provides no rules other than the aggregation of utility. Nothing is forbidden if it increases aggregate utility. When added to the uncertainty about how to determine what is good and how achieving that good is to be measured, lack of definition about means renders the application of utilitarianism to understanding health care equity as social justice minimally, if at all, useful.

Socialism and Communism

The global struggle between capitalism and communism was arguably the most important political phenomenon of the 20th century. So, the relevance of communism to a discussion of visions of social justice is beyond doubt. Also, socialism remains a major political philosophy affecting the discourse about health care equity, here and in other countries. For example, in many Western industrialized countries, health care is a governmental service offered as part of the state social contract with the citizens.

Communist philosophy envisions the abolition (through class struggle) of the divide between individual and community interests, indeed between those of the individual and the species, and the rise of a corresponding ethos free of greed and envy—from each according to their ability, to each according to their need—an ethos of true equity based on advanced technology maximizing the effective use of the world's resources (Singer, 1980). In such a world, the state as an armed force to do policing and fight wars would be unnecessary and would "wither away."

Equity is paramount, at least in principle or aspiration. All have equal access to social and economic resources, and, therefore, the opportunity for equitable outcomes. As applied to health equity, it would mean focusing on consistency of health-promoting and health care systems, as well as provision of care as needed, not based on privilege or standing.

Socialism is a political philosophy that has been defined in varying ways over time and place, and carries different connotations in different historical contexts.

Socialism usually refers to a political theory of social organization that advocates that the means of production, distribution, and exchange should be owned or regulated by the community as a whole. Thus, health care and health management within a range of socialistic perspectives can be state owned and managed or could be private or a mix of private and state, but with ultimate regulation and determination of goals in regard to equity under the control of the state (representing the community as a whole).

Today, it is common to refer to the health care systems of a number of capitalist nation-states, particularly in Europe, as socialist because of the high level of state support for health care and social welfare. What seems accurate and particularly relevant to perspectives and models of health equity and related social justice in this country is the viewing of commodification of health care as inappropriate or contrary to justice (Pellegrino, 1999). This is similar to how various institutions in our country, such as public education, roadways, fire and police protection, and air and water safety, function and are viewed as something one's access to is independent of economic or political standing. As there are many who think that health equity rests on movement to a single-payer state-supported approach, the implications of this philosophy for the means and ends related to health equity deserve careful consideration. Most fundamentally, it is the assumption that health care should not be a matter of personal economic exchange, but seen as a right of membership in society, with equity in access and quality as fundamental to social justice.

CONCLUSION

As the discourse about health equity and its relation to social justice proceeds, it seems valuable to consider the implications of philosophical roots of some of the competing ideologies and positions regarding equity and social justice. Recognizing the relevance of various cultural approaches to balancing societal and individual needs can only make our deliberations more transparent, lucid, and powerful and, therefore, strengthen democracy. Acknowledging these approaches can advance our understanding of ways to address and apply diverse values as well as clarify the implications of different policy ideas.

As we have attempted to delineate briefly, a major distinction between philosophies and related definitions of health equity and strategies to achieve it is the extent to which society values individual freedom and choice over group well-being. A closely related distinction is the relative emphasis on broad and even access to resources versus variation related to choice or personal capabilities. A third major consideration is the role of the government in managing the means to equity and in ensuring its realization.

While the dominant political ideology in America today is liberalism, we have recently seen a range of popular variants from Donald Trump's populism to Bernie Sanders's socialism. There are many different interpretations of liberal ideology in health equity and social-justice discourse and multiple other philosophies that are relevant. In working to develop coherent policy based on social justice or equity, it can only help to draw on as wide as possible a range of human wisdom as we can.

As the question of how to overcome and rid our society of inequities due to discrimination and other historical legacies in health, perhaps more careful consideration is needed of what is meant by equity, how that relates to concepts of justice, and how that translates to policy and action. How can innovative policies drawing on a wide range of cultural and philosophical traditions improve our discourse while fitting practically into our existing social and political context? How might research help determine which approaches to equity in health opportunities, access to care, quality of care, and life quality and longevity actually will provide improvements by bringing the status of disadvantaged groups up to that of the more privileged and thereby realize social justice?

REFERENCES

Braveman, P. 2006. Health disparities and health equity: concepts and measurement. *Annual Review of Public Health* 27:167–194.

Buchanan, A. 1984. The right to a decent minimum of health care. *Philosophy and Public Affairs* 13:55–78.

Daniels, N. 1985. *Just health care*. New York: Oxford University Press.

Hanh, T. N. 2006. We have the compassion and understanding necessary to heal the world: 2003 speech to the U.S. Congress. In *Mindful politics: A Buddhist guide to making the world a better place*. Boston: Wisdom Publications, 129–138.

Ling, T. 1993. *The Buddha's philosophy of man*. London: Everyman's Library.

Mukenge, T. 2002. *Culture and customs of the Congo*. Westport, CT: Greenwood Press.

Nussbaum, M. C. 2007. *Frontiers of justice*. Cambridge, MA: Harvard University Press.

Pellegrino, E. D. 1999. The commodification of medical and health care: The moral consequences of a paradigm shift from a professional to a market ethic. *Journal of Medical Philosophy* 24:243–266.

Rand, A. 1961. *The virtue of selfishness*. New York: Signet.

Rawls, J. 1971. *A theory of justice*. Cambridge, MA: Belknap.

Rosemont, H. 1991. *A Chinese mirror: Moral reflections on political economy and society*. La Salle, IL: Open Court Publishing.

Ruger, J. P. 2010. *Health and social justice*. Oxford, United Kingdom: Oxford University Press.

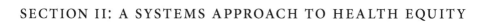

SECTION II: A SYSTEMS APPROACH TO HEALTH EQUITY

6

EXPULSION AND SUSPENSION IN EARLY EDUCATION AS MATTERS OF SOCIAL JUSTICE AND HEALTH EQUITY

Shantel E. Meek, PhD, and Walter S. Gilliam, PhD

Scientists have a central role in addressing the challenges that face society. The primary purpose of research should be to inform policies and practices that address serious problems in our nation and world. Today, in America, we have an alarming issue that is lacking in both basic and applied research—the "preschool-to-prison pipeline," a now familiar phrase that describes the disturbing trend of setting children—disproportionately children of color—on a trajectory toward the criminal justice system through practices such as early expulsion and suspension.

Though there is a body of literature on the school-to-prison pipeline, including some research on the associated mental and behavioral health status of the caregivers and early education teachers expelling young children and the sometimes traumatic experiences of the child leading to certain behaviors, we need more and better research on the entry point during preschool. Why are expulsions and suspensions happening in early childhood settings with children as young as 2 years old? What are the long-term consequences for these children? And, most important, how can they be prevented? We cannot address the preschool-to-prison pipeline if we ignore the earliest entry point. This paper addresses what is known and not yet known about early childhood expulsions and suspensions, specifically focusing on the disproportionate application of these exclusionary sanctions to our youngest children, and offers suggestions for future directions in research.

Early childhood expulsions and suspensions are matters of health and education equity. As discussed later in this paper, access to high-quality early education has been shown to be related to a vast array of positive benefits, especially for children from low-income families; yet children of color who are low income are less likely to gain access to high-quality early education programs and are more likely to attend poorly resourced programs that provide them, their families, and the staff who work in these programs fewer supportive practices and services that bolster behavioral and mental health that are necessary to ensure that children are on a positive trajectory to succeed in school and life.

Starting as young as infancy and toddlerhood, children of color are at highest risk for being expelled from early care and education programs. Early expulsions and suspensions lead to greater gaps in access to resources for young children and thus create increasing gaps in later achievement and well-being. Early education programs are a main source of referral to additional services and supports, such as mental health supports or early intervention. By being expelled from the system, children are not only losing access to their early learning experiences, but they may also be less likely to be referred to—and receive—the services and supports they need to thrive. These disparities in access to resources start early and may compound over time. Research indicates that early expulsions and suspensions predict later expulsions and suspensions, academic failure, school dropout, and an increased likelihood of later incarceration—a "preschool-to-prison pipeline," or perhaps "cradle-to-prison pipeline," with devastating and costly consequences.

Social justice—equal access and opportunity for all—has been a core American value since our founding as a nation. That value, however, is not fully realized in the lives of millions of our citizens, people of color, recent immigrants, individuals with disabilities, people who are low income, and others, nor has it ever been. The fact that racial, ethnic, socioeconomic, and ability-based disparities and inequities are widespread across most aspects of society is not surprising to most. Indeed, millions of Americans live these inequities each day. Yet, the fact that these disparities start early, perhaps before birth, and are pervasive throughout children's lives before they even enter kindergarten is still surprising to many. A serious discussion about social justice and health equity in America must start with reflection on the opportunities and access to resources we offer, and do not offer, our youngest children, especially those from historically marginalized communities.

DISPARITIES IN ACCESS

The beginning years of any child's life are critical for building the early foundation needed for healthy developmental trajectories and success in school and later life. During this period, the brain develops at a pace unlike any other and is extraordinarily sensitive to and affected by children's environments, experiences, and relationships. Those formative first 5 years are simultaneously the most opportune and vulnerable for setting children on a trajectory for success or failure. There is a robust literature indicating that early adversities can set the stage for later adversities. Unfortunately, these early adversities are all too common, and supports to buffer children from these adversities are not common enough. High-quality early care and education programs for children birth through 4 years old have been shown to produce meaningful positive impacts in the lives of young children, especially for children of low-income families dealing with the stressors and lack of enrichment opportunities that all too often accompany financial disadvantage (Pianta et al., 2009).

Unfortunately, the positive supports provided by high-quality early education are often inequitably distributed. Low-income children and children of color alike have less access to high-quality, early-learning programs, except Head Start (Barnett et al., 2013). They are overrepresented in unlicensed and unregulated childcare settings and are more likely to attend lower-quality and underresourced preschool programs and elementary and secondary schools (Hanushek and Rivkin, 2006). Insufficiently resourced programs often lack appropriate compensation and adequate supportive services for their staff—such as health benefits, mental health supports, and paid sick days (Whitebook et al., 2016). In addition, low-resourced programs are more likely to be in low-income communities where staff face many of the same stressors as the families who use their services, including food and housing insecurity, unsafe communities, and lack of health resources. Evidence shows that unmet health and mental health needs in early childhood education staff, such as depression and severe job stress, negatively affect the ways educators interact with children (IOM and NRC, 2012).

For those low-income children and children of color who do gain access to an early childhood program, they are more likely to be pushed out through exclusionary practices such as suspension and expulsion. This is particularly true for young African American boys (Department of Education, 2014; Gilliam, 2005). Low-income children and children of color have less "front door" access to high-quality, early-learning programs, and they are also pushed out the "back door" in these settings at disproportionate rates.

This "push out" phenomenon has become of increasing concern to the early childhood field over the past several years. In 2005, the first nationally representative study to examine the issue found that expulsion and suspension rates were three or more times higher in early childhood settings than in K-12 settings, with boys being expelled at 4.5 times the rate of girls and African American preschoolers expelled at twice the rate of others (Gilliam, 2005). Recent findings from the Department of Education (2016) indicate that the racial disparities in suspensions from school-based prekindergarten settings are perhaps even more alarming than previously thought. African American preschoolers were found to be 3.6 times as likely to receive one or more suspensions as white preschoolers. While African American children make up 19 percent of preschool enrollment, they comprise 47 percent of preschoolers suspended one or more times. Similarly, boys were 3.0 times as likely as girls to be suspended one or more times. African American boys represent 19 percent of the male preschool enrollment, but 45 percent of male preschool children receive one or more out-of-school suspensions. African American girls represent 20 percent of the female preschool enrollment, but 54 percent of female preschool children receive one or more out-of-school suspensions. These rates and disparities are similar to those reported 2 years earlier (Department of Education, 2014).

These figures have serious implications. Early expulsion and suspension predict later expulsion and suspension, and students who are expelled or suspended from school are as much as 10 times more likely to drop out of high school, experience academic failure and grade retention, hold negative school attitudes, and face incarceration than those who are not (APA, 2008; Council on School Health, 2013; Petras et al., 2011). Taken together, these disturbing trends suggest that the school-to-prison pipeline has an entry point long before the first day of kindergarten, and the implications span economic, educational, and health outcomes.

Fortunately, in the past 2 years, federal, state, and municipal governments have sought to eliminate preschool expulsions and suspensions. President Obama's My Brother's Keeper initiative, which seeks to increase life-span opportunities and equity for all children, including boys and young men of color, highlighted eliminating expulsion and suspension from early learning settings and addressing disparities in these practices as key recommendations in its strategy (White House, 2014). Related federal efforts include a December 2014 joint departmental statement of the Department of Health and Human Services and the Department of Education (HHS and ED, 2014), calling for the elimination of preschool expulsion and suspension, as well as implementation of early childhood disciplinary policies that are free of bias and discrimination. This federal position has been endorsed by over 30 of the nation's largest and most visible professional organizations serving young children (Standing Together, 2016). Also, rule changes to the federal Head Start Performance Standards (Administration for Children and Families, 2015) seek to "prohibit or severely limit" suspensions and "explicitly prohibit" expulsions in all Head Start programs, as well as require programs to engage a mental health consultant, collaborate with parents, use appropriate community resources, and address potential bias in disciplinary decisions. HHS and ED have also invested in training and technical assistance to support early childhood programs and educators in eliminating expulsions and suspensions.

HHS established the first National Center of Excellence for Infant and Early Childhood Mental Health Consultation (ECMHC), which will develop new resources and provide intensive technical assistance to tribal communities and states on building sustainable ECMHC systems. HHS and ED also funded the Technical Assistance Center on Positive Behavior Intervention and Supports to implement the Pyramid Equity Project, which will develop and disseminate resources that support children's social-emotional and behavioral development and build the capacity of early educators in implementing culturally responsive practices and addressing implicit bias. States and local communities around the country have also begun addressing the issue by passing laws and policies that severely limit or ban early childhood expulsion and suspension practices (e.g., Arkansas, Connecticut, Chicago Public Schools, District of Columbia, New York City Public Schools) or expand support for early childhood mental health consultation (e.g., Arkansas, Colorado, Connecticut, Ohio; Administration for Children and Families, 2016). It is clear, however, that more needs to be done by all parties, including establishing policies that prohibit expulsion across program types and settings and fully expanding social-emotional supports for early educators and early childhood mental health services to meet need.

SOCIAL JUSTICE AND CIVIL RIGHTS

The proliferation of early care and education programs in the United States has been largely supported by developmental science documenting many positive educational and later-life outcomes associated with attendance (Pianta et al., 2009). Many of these positive outcomes are monetarily quantifiable (e.g., reductions in grade retention, school dropout, and later incarceration, as well as increases in lifetime earnings and home ownership which result in increased tax payments), allowing economists to estimate the economic return on investment provided by early education. Recently, the White House Council of Economic Advisors (2014) calculated that, for every dollar spent on early education initiatives, society would receive a return on investment of $8.60. They further report that enabling all families to enroll their children in early education at the same rate as that of affluent families would result in billions in earnings contributed to the economy, and translate to an increase in GDP of 0.16 to 0.44 percent.

To a large degree this science is based on economic impact analyses from three longitudinal evaluations of early education—the Perry Preschool Study (Schweinhart et al., 2005), the Abecedarian Study (Campbell, 1994), and the Chicago Child-Parent Centers Study (Reynolds et al., 2011). These are three of the most widely cited studies on the economic benefits of high-quality early education, and each of these studies shows remarkable returns on investment. It is also true that each of these studies was conducted with samples that were overwhelmingly African American—100 percent for the Perry Preschool Study, 98 percent for the Abecedarian Study, and 93 percent for the Chicago Child-Parent Centers Study. Racial disparities in expulsions and suspensions in early education pose at least two major challenges. First, disparities in these exclusionary measures may present a serious undermining of the return on investment potential for early education, because the children being excluded are disproportionately the ones for whom we have the most evidence of favorable economic returns. Second, racial disparities in expulsions from early education create a serious and disturbing ethical, moral, and civil rights problem in that the children whose data were used to purchase the political will to fund early education for American children of all races are disproportionately the ones later denied access. Clearly, there is no reasonable angle by which racial disparities on expulsion and suspension from American early education programs should be tolerated.

Expulsion and suspension are by-products of inequities and challenges in the early education system and broader society. These forms of early exclusion are pivotal points of influence in young children's lives that must be addressed by a broad coalition of stakeholders, including researchers; policy makers; and local districts, schools, and community-based programs. The research community must actively engage in conducting and translating research in this area. Though there is some research on early expulsion and suspension, there remain large gaps in many areas, including longitudinal studies documenting the long-term sequelae of early disciplinary exclusions and rigorous evaluations of interventions designed to prevent these exclusions. Much of our knowledge is taken from research conducted in the K-12 educational system. Although this research has relevance to the early education system, K-12 and early education are very different systems in terms of the developmental needs of the students and the ways the systems are structured.

THE RATE AND CAUSES OF EARLY CHILDHOOD EXPULSIONS AND SUSPENSIONS

The three main early education programs in the United States are Head Start and Early Head Start, which serve about 1 million children birth to age 5 each year; state prekindergarten, which serves about 1.3 million 3- and 4-year-olds each year; and childcare, which serves nearly 11 million children under age 5 or about 63 percent of the nation's children in this age group (Laughlin, 2013).[1] Funding levels, quality, infrastructure, eligibility, services, data systems, workforce, and affordability vary greatly between each of these sectors; for pre-kindergarten and childcare, the differences are often great across state, county, and municipal lines.

Given the tremendous variability in early education programs, it is not surprising that we do not have an estimate of the overall national rate of disciplinary exclusions in the early years across all early education settings. Estimates have been largely isolated to one or another part of the early education system or to specific parts of the country. Available research, however, suggests that rates are much higher than expected, and by some estimates they are much higher than in K-12. For example, a nationally representative study published in 2005 found that over 10 percent of teachers in *state-funded prekindergarten programs* reported expelling at least one preschooler in the past year (Gilliam, 2005). A 2006 study examined expulsion in *childcare programs in Massachusetts* and found that 39 percent of teachers reported expelling a child in the past year (Gilliam and Shahar, 2006). An unpublished survey of childcare providers in Detroit, Michigan, found rates similar to those in Massachusetts (Grannan et al., 1999). Even infants and toddlers are at high risk for childcare expulsion, with 42 percent of infant/toddler childcare centers across Illinois reporting at least one expulsion in the past year (Cutler and Gilkerson, 2002). Taken together, annual expulsions in state-funded prekindergartens are estimated to be about 3 times higher than in K-12, and in childcare programs, many of which are less regulated, more poorly resourced, and have a less trained workforce, it is as much as 13 times higher.

Turning to suspension, recent data from the Department of Education indicate that 6 percent of *school districts with preschool programs* reported suspending at least one preschool child from public-school prekindergartens during the 2011–2012 academic year. Although providing an incomplete picture of the broader early education system, these numbers are alarming enough to prompt immediate action. While states and communities begin to address this issue in policy and practice, it is critical that researchers and policy makers collaborate to collect the appropriate data and provide a more complete analysis of expulsion and suspension rates across the early childhood system.

Researchers have not yet fully examined the sources of these high suspension and expulsions rates, though correlational analyses have provided some promising directions and hypotheses. One study found that higher rates of expulsion were associated with higher reports of teachers' stress and depression, larger "classroom" sizes, and less access to mental health consultants and other support systems (Gilliam and Shahar, 2006). Also, early childhood rates may be high because early care and education are voluntary, whereas in most K-12 grades, school attendance is compulsory, and thus expulsion and suspension are usually not legal matters in the early years. Because preschool attendance is not legally mandated and expulsions typically have no legal implications, the procedures for expelling a student appear to follow no due process guidelines and may be more informal in nature. In addition, most early childhood programs do not have established policies against expulsion and suspension and many programs do not have the resources to support their workforce in appropriately managing large teacher–child ratios and group sizes, developmentally typical challenging behavior, and children who may need additional supports (e.g., early intervention, health or mental health services). Empirically identifying the contributors to early expulsion and suspension will enable researchers and policy makers to target investments and interventions more precisely and effectively.

GENDER AND RACE DISPARITIES IN EARLY CHILDHOOD EXPULSIONS AND SUSPENSIONS

As noted, there are large racial disparities in expulsion and suspension in the early years, similar to trends documented in K-12 settings, with young African American boys being expelled and suspended at significantly higher rates than their peers. Again, the *why* has not yet been addressed by early childhood research, but studies demonstrating similar disparities in K-12 students have found that potential contributors may include uneven or biased implementation of disciplinary policies, discriminatory discipline practices, school racial climate, underresourced programs, and inadequate education and training for teachers, especially in self-reflective strategies to identify and correct potential biases in perceptions and practice (Gilliam, 2005; Gregory et al., 2010). Relative to their white peers, African American elementary students are more than twice as likely to be referred to the principal's office for challenging behaviors and significantly more likely to be expelled or suspended, even when the behavioral infractions are similar (Skiba et al., 2011). These racial disparities are independent of socioeconomic status, suggesting that race is a stronger driver for disciplinary disparities than the economic challenges that are often associated with race (Skiba et al., 2002).

Gender and race disparities in early expulsions and suspensions may also be associated with several factors related to stress tolerance and access to high-quality early learning environments and supports. Regarding gender, boys appear to be more susceptible than girls to the ill effects of poverty, trauma, stressed communities, and low-quality schools, with the results being a greater likelihood for truancy, poor academic achievement, behavioral problems, school dropout, and crime (Autor et al., 2015). Even when the degree of stress and the amount of familial supports are the same, boys tend to show more adverse reaction than their sisters (Bertrand and Pan, 2011). As mentioned earlier, children of color and children from low-income families have less access to high-quality early learning programs (Barnett et al., 2013; Hanushek and Rivkin, 2006). They are overrepresented in unlicensed and unregulated childcare settings and are more likely to attend lower-quality and underresourced preschool programs and elementary and secondary schools (Hanushek and Rivkin, 2006).

POTENTIAL ROLE OF IMPLICIT BIASES

A report from the American Psychological Association's Task Force on Preventing Discrimination and Promoting Diversity found that biases—including implicit biases—are pervasive across people and institutions (Jones et al., 2012), though this phenomenon has been more carefully examined in some aspects of society, such as the criminal justice and health systems, than others. One potential contributor of race and gender disparities in early childhood expulsions and suspensions is implicit biases regarding how teachers, administrators, and other staff perceive and appraise classroom behaviors. Expulsions and suspensions are not child behaviors; they are adult decisions. Although the behaviors of children may impact adult decision-making processes, implicit biases about boys and children of color may impact how those behaviors are perceived and how they are addressed.

Though there is little research examining this phenomenon in early childhood settings, studies of school-age children have identified disturbing trends. In a recent study, researchers presented schoolteachers with two fictional student disciplinary records (Okonofua and Eberhardt, 2015). The records were randomly labeled with either stereotypical African American names or stereotypical white names. Both fictional students had engaged in minor school violations (e.g., classroom disturbance). Teachers reported that they felt more "troubled" by the offenses of the African American student and were more likely to recommend severe punishment for the African American student after the second infraction, including suspension, compared to the white student with the same record. They were also asked how certain they were of the child's race. Those who reported being more certain were more likely to label the African American child as a "troublemaker" and report that his or her behavior was part of a pattern, as opposed to a single occurrence. Another study found that university undergraduate students given a vignette of a child with a challenging behavior that was randomly associated with pictures of children of different races rated African American children as young as age 10 years old as being significantly less innocent and more culpable (Goff et al., 2014). They also estimated that the

African American children in the pictures were on average 4.5 years older than they really were. A major predictor of a teacher's plans to expel a preschooler is the degree to which that teacher feels the child may pose a danger to the other children (Gilliam and Reyes, 2016). Therefore, the degree to which African American children are perceived as more culpable or older than they really are may have significant implications for race disparities in expulsion rates.

These tendencies to view child behaviors differentially based on the race of the child may be a manifestation of more generalized implicit biases regarding race and criminal or delinquent behavior. For example, in a series of studies with police officers and college students, participants were more likely to direct their eye gaze toward African American faces as opposed to white faces whenever the experimenters invoked concepts of crime or delinquency (Eberhardt et al., 2004). This automatic association between race and perceived threat of aggression has been shown even when the African American face shown was that of a 5-year-old boy (Todd et al., 2016). Implicit biases such as these may be related to differential application of empathy learned at a young age, as was demonstrated in a study that found that 7- and 10-year-olds rated African American children as feeling significantly less pain from injuries such as hitting their heads or biting their tongues, relative to white children (Dore et al., 2014). This dehumanizing tendency to view African American children as less susceptible to pain may make it easier to also view them as more culpable or guilty by removing the moderating effects of empathy.

Biases in expectations may also influence which children teachers feel are most likely to pose significant classroom behavioral challenges. In one study, white middle school and high school English teachers were each provided a poorly written essay to grade. The student name on the essay was randomized to suggest it was authored by either an African American, a white, or a Latino student. Students of color were assigned significantly higher grades. This "positive feedback bias" suggested that teachers may have been demonstrating biases in their expectations, whereby African American and Latino students were expected to be capable of only lower-quality essays and are therefore given a higher grade, while white students are expected to write better essays and are thereby given a lower grade (Harber et al., 2012). A robust scientific literature exists regarding these "shifting standards," where people are held to differing standards based on deeply held gender and racial stereotypes regarding their expected capabilities (Biernat, 2003). These shifting-standards biases also may be present in early childhood settings and regarding child behaviors, and future research is needed to explore this potential. If such biases in expectations or standards exist, they may lead teachers to more closely scrutinize the behaviors of some children relative to others or may lead to decreased behavioral expectations that can later become self-fulfilling.

Combined, these studies may provide some insights on the context surrounding expulsions and suspensions in early childhood settings, but more direct analyses are necessary to fully understand the issue and the many likely contributory factors. Understanding the degree to which implicit biases may contribute to expulsion and suspension decisions by early education staff and administrators is an important step to a fuller understanding of the source of disciplinary dispari-ties. Follow-up questions would include whether factors such as teacher depres-sion or job stress or large group sizes and child–teacher ratios may exasperate existing implicit biases, and whether better teacher–parent communication and classroom-level supports may mitigate the effects of implicit biases.

CALL TO ACTION FOR THE RESEARCH FIELD

Research on the consequences of expulsion and suspension from the K-12 system and data that suggest that these harmful practices may be happening at higher rates in the years before kindergarten are cause for action. While policy makers and practitioners are responding to these immediate needs, researchers must help fill the knowledge gaps that are preventing faster and more effective progress. The following research directions would help inform policy and investment decisions in this important area.

The medium- and long-term consequences of expulsion and suspension from early childhood settings have not been studied. In fact, there have been no longitudinal studies looking at this issue, starting in the early childhood years. Research on exclusionary discipline in the K-12 system indicates that suspension and expulsion from school can influence a number of adverse outcomes across development, health, and education. As previously mentioned, young students who are expelled or suspended are as much as 10 times more likely to drop out of high school, experience academic failure and grade retention, hold negative school attitudes, and face incarceration. Research also indicates that expulsion and suspension early in a child's educational trajectory predicts expulsion and suspension later (Raffaele-Mendez, 2003). What becomes of these expelled pre-schoolers? Do they then move to other early care and education settings, as their parents need care to support their employment, only to be expelled again? Do they move to less regulated and lower-quality settings or informal settings that do not have the tools to support children's development? Early expulsions and suspensions may have additional adverse consequences such as hindering social-emotional and behavioral development; delaying or interfering with the process of identifying and addressing underlying issues, which may include exposure to trauma, developmental delays or disabilities, or mental health issues; negatively impacting parents' views on both their young children's potential and schools as a safe and accepting place; and causing added family stress and burden, the effects of which are felt by young children (Van Egeren et al., 2011). Future research should focus on better understanding the medium- and long-term consequences of expulsions and suspension in early care and education programs.

In order to create more effective methods for preventing early childhood expulsions and suspensions, more needs to be understood regarding the processes by which young children are identified for these exclusionary disciplines. How do teachers and administrators make these determinations? Would clearer policies and procedures in early care and education settings reduce incidence rates? Would they narrow disparities in these practices? In what ways might better teacher–family relationships serve as a preventive? In addition, it will be important for researchers to understand the differences and relationships between expulsions and suspensions. Do suspensions mask expulsions? That is, does a program suspending a child for an extended period of time force the family to find alternative placement and leave the program? Given that the terms "expulsion" and "suspensions" are not always the terms used in early childhood systems for dismissing a child from a program due to behavior, researchers should be thoughtful regarding how they ask questions and collect data on this issue.

At present, no studies have been published regarding the potential for implicit bias in how preschool and childcare teachers appraise and detect challenging behaviors in young children, and more specifically how implicit bias may account for the increased risk of expulsion and suspension in preschool boys and African American children. Nonetheless, recent research suggests that implicit bias may be reduced through interventions designed to address biases directly (Devine et al., 2012; Jones et al., 2012; van Nunspeet et al., 2015), raising the question of whether evidence-based, bias-reducing interventions should be a core component of ongoing early childhood teacher training. Also, clear guiding principles by which early educators may explore and discover their own implicit biases and strive to deliver more equitable services may be a useful tool (St. John et al., 2012). How can the negative impacts of implicit bias be understood and reduced in early care and education settings? Increased attention to evidence-based interventions and approaches that prevent expulsion, suspension, and other exclusionary discipline practices, including ECMHC and positive behavior intervention and supports (PBIS), was one of the primary aims of the 2014 HHS and ED joint position statement. These approaches are further encouraged through language included in the reauthorized Child Care and Development Block Grant Act of

2014,[2] the federal law that helps working families receive public assistance for childcare in the United States, as well as national best-practices guidelines for childcare centers (American Academy of Pediatrics and American Public Health Association, 2013). Further, all Head Start programs are required to support children's social-emotional development and ensure access to an early childhood mental health consultant for children and families in the program.

ECMHC is a multilevel preventive intervention that teams mental health professionals with early childhood education staff to improve the social-emotional and behavioral health and development of young children through better teacher–child and teacher–family interactions. Research suggests that ECMHC may be effective in increasing children's social skills; reducing children's challenging behavior; preventing preschool suspensions and expulsions; improving child–adult relationships; decreasing teacher job stress, burnout, and turnover; and identifying child concerns early, so that children get the supports they need as soon as possible (Hepburn et al., 2013). Early childhood teachers who report regular access to mental health consultants are half as likely to report expelling a young child than teachers who report no such access (Gilliam, 2005). Though several ECMHC models have been evaluated with each demonstrating positive associations on children's outcomes, only Connecticut's Early Childhood Partnership Program, a manualized and replicable form of ECMHC, has been evaluated in randomized controlled evaluations demonstrating positive effects on child behaviors (Gilliam et al., 2016). The early childhood model of PBIS, called the pyramid model, has also shown promising results in supporting children's social-emotional development and reducing challenging behaviors. A randomized controlled study examining the pyramid model in early childhood settings found that children enrolled in the intervention classrooms demonstrated improved social skills and reductions in problem behavior, compared to control classrooms (Hemmeter et al., 2016).

Further rigorous experimental evaluations are needed on both ECMHC and PBIS to further validate these promising approaches, given that only one published or in-press, randomized controlled evaluation exists for each. Given the urgency of the need for interventions that address this issue, rapid-cycle evaluation approaches that can provide valid data to policy makers and program leaders faster on the efficacy of these and similar models should also be considered. Specifically, these and similar models should be evaluated regarding their long-term impacts on teacher and child behaviors and interactions, exclusionary discipline practices, and whether and how these interventions address racial and gender disparities. Enhancements to these models that directly target disproportionality, including by addressing issues surrounding implicit bias, should also be evaluated.

Research regarding the rates and disparities in early childhood expulsions and suspensions is only a beginning. Now that the problem has been highlighted and potential policy directions identified, more specific research is needed to better understand the determinants and the effective models to prevent and eventually eliminate early childhood expulsions and suspensions for all of our young children in all of our early care and education settings. The recommendations noted would go far in terms of moving us from awareness of the problem toward solutions for ending the preschool-to-prison pipeline by providing all of our young children a more equitable start at fulfilling their potentials.

ENDNOTES

1. Additionally, over 350,000 children ages birth to 3 years with disabilities or developmental delays are provided federal- and state-funded early intervention services, and over 145,000 young children and families are provided services through the Federal Home Visiting Program. Both programs also have the goal of supporting healthy early childhood development.
2. S. 1086, 113 Cong., 2d sess. Available from https://www.congress.gov/113/bills/s1086/BILLS-113s1086enr.pdf.

REFERENCES

Administration for Children and Families. 2015. Head Start performance standards, notice of proposed rulemaking [section 1302.17: Suspension and Expulsion]. *Federal Register* 80(118). Available from https://www.gpo.gov/fdsys/pkg/FR-2015-06-19/pdf/2015-14379.pdf.

Administration for Children and Families. 2016. *State and local action to prevent expulsion and suspension in early learning settings: Spotlighting progress in policy and supports.* Available from https://www.acf.hhs.gov/sites/default/files/ecd/state_and_local_profiles_expulsion.pdf.

American Academy of Pediatrics and American Public Health Association. 2013. *Stepping stones to caring for our children: National health and safety performance standards; Guidelines for early care and education programs,* 3rd ed. Washington, DC: Author. Available from http://nrckids.org/index.cfm/products/stepping-stones-to-caring-for-our-children-3rd-edition-ss3/stepping-stones-to-caring-for-our-children-3rd-edition-ss3/.

APA (American Psychological Association). 2008. *Zero Tolerance Task Force report: An evidentiary review and recommendations.* Washington, DC: Author.

Autor, D., D. Figlio, K. Karbownik, J. Roth, and M. Wasserman. 2015. *Family disadvantage and the gender gap in behavioral and educational outcomes.* Working Paper Series 15–16. Evanston, IL: Institute for Policy Research, Northwestern University.

Barnett, S., M. Carolan, and D. Johns. 2013. *Equity and excellence: African American children's access to quality preschool.* New Brunswick, NJ: National Institute for Early Education Research. Available from http://nieer.org/sites/nieer/files/Equity%20

and%20Excellence%20African-American%20Children%E2%80%99s%20Access%20 to%20Quality%20Preschool_0.pdf.

Bertrand, M., and J. Pan. 2011. *The trouble with boys: Social influences and the gender gap in disruptive behavior.* NBER Working Paper No. 17541. Cambridge, MA: National Bureau of Economic Research.

Biernat, M. 2003. Toward a broader view of social stereotyping. *American Psychologist* 58:1019–1027.

Campbell, F. A. 1994. Effects of early intervention on intellectual and academic achievement: A follow-up study of children from low-income families. *Child Development* 65:684–698.

Council on School Health. 2013. Out-of-school suspension and expulsion. *Pediatrics* 131(3):e1000–e1007.

Cutler, A., and L. Gilkerson. 2002. *Unmet needs project: A research, coalition building and policy initiative on the unmet needs of infants, toddlers and families.* Chicago, IL: University of Illinois at Chicago and Erikson Institute.

Department of Education, Office of Civil Rights. 2014. *Data snapshot: Early childhood education. Civil rights data collection.* Issue brief #2. Available from https://www2. ed.gov/about/offices/list/ocr/docs/crdc-early-learning-snapshot.pdf.

Department of Education, Office of Civil Rights. 2016. *2013–2014 Civil rights data collection: Key data highlights on equity and opportunity gaps in our nation's public schools.* Available from http://www2.ed.gov/about/offices/list/ocr/docs/crdc-2013-14.html.

Devine, P. G., P. S. Forscher, A. J. Austin, and W. T. L. Cox. 2012. Long-term reduction in implicit race bias: A prejudice habit-breaking intervention. *Journal of Experimental Social Psychology* 48:1267–1278.

Dore, R., K. Hoffman, A. Lillard, and S. Trawalter. 2014. Children's racial bias in perceptions of others' pain. *British Journal of Developmental Psychology* 32:218–231.

Eberhardt, J. L., P. A. Goff, V. J. Purdie, and P. G. Davies. 2004. Seeing black: Race, crime, and visual processing. *Journal of Personality and Social Psychology* 87:876–893.

Gilliam, W. S. 2005. *Prekindergarteners left behind: Expulsion rates in state prekindergarten systems.* New Haven, CT: Yale University Child Study Center. Available from http://www.ziglercenter.yale.edu/publications/National%20Prek%20Study_expulsion_tcm350-34774_tcm350-284-32.pdf.

Gilliam, W. S., and G. Shahar. 2006. Prekindergarten expulsion and suspension: Rates and predictors in one state. *Infants and Young Children* 19:228–245.

Gilliam, W. S., and C. Reyes. 2016. *Teacher decision-making factors that lead to preschool expulsion: Scale development and preliminary validation of the preschool expulsion risk measure.* Manuscript submitted for review.

Gilliam, W. S., A. N. Maupin, and C. R. Reyes. 2016. Early childhood mental health consultation: Results of a statewide random-controlled evaluation. *Journal of the American Academy of Child and Adolescent Psychiatry* 55:754–761.

Goff, P. A., M. C. Jackson, B. Allison, L. Di Leone, M. Culotta, and N. A. DiTomasso. 2014. The essence of innocence: Consequences of dehumanizing black children. *Journal of Personality and Social Psychology* 106:526–545.

Grannan, M., C. Carlier, and C. E. Cole. 1999. *Early childhood care and education expulsion prevention project*. Southgate, MI: Downriver Guidance Clinic, Department of Early Childhood Programs.

Gregory, A., R. J. Skiba, and P. A. Noguera. 2010. The achievement gap and the discipline gap: Two sides of the same coin? *Educational Researcher* 39(1):59–68.

Hanushek, E. A., and S. G. Rivkin. 2006. *School quality and the black-white achievement gap*. NBER Working Paper No. 12651. Cambridge, MA: National Bureau of Economic Research.

Harber, K. D., J. L. Gorman, F. P. Gengaro, S. Butisingh, W. Tsang, and R. Ouellette. 2012. Students' race and teachers' social support affect the positive feedback bias in public schools. *Journal of Educational Psychology* 104:1149–1161.

Hemmeter, M. L., P. A. Snyder, L. Fox, and J. Algina. 2016. Evaluating the implementation of the pyramid model for promoting social-emotional competence in early childhood classrooms. *Topics in Early Childhood Special Education* 36:133–146.

Hepburn, K. S., D. F. Perry, E. M. Shivers, and W. S. Gilliam. 2013. Early childhood mental health consultation as an evidence-based practice: Where does it stand? *Zero to Three* 33(5):10–19.

HHS and ED (Department of Health and Human Services and Department of Education). 2014. *Policy statement on expulsion and suspension policies in early childhood settings*. Available from https://www.acf.hhs.gov/sites/default/files/ecd/expulsion_suspension_final.pdf.

IOM and NRC (Institute of Medicine and National Research Council). 2012. *The early childhood care and education workforce: Challenges and opportunities: A workshop report*. Washington, DC: The National Academies Press.

Jones, J. M., S. D. Cochran, M. Fine, S. Gaertner, R. Mendoza-Denton, M. Shih, and D. W. Sue. 2012. *Dual pathways to a better America: Preventing discrimination and promoting diversity*. Washington, DC: American Psychological Association, Presidential Task Force on Preventing Discrimination and Promoting Diversity. Available from https://www.apa.org/pubs/info/reports/dual-pathways-report.pdf.

Laughlin, L. 2013. *Who's minding the kids? Child care arrangements: Spring 2011*. Current Population Reports, P70-135. Washington, DC: U.S. Census Bureau. Available from https://www.census.gov/prod/2013pubs/p70-135.pdf.

Okonofua, J. A., and J. L. Eberhardt. 2015. Two strikes: Race and the disciplining of young students. *Psychological Science* 26:617–624.

Petras, H., K. E. Masyn, J. A., Buckley, N. S., Ialongo, and S. Kellam, 2011. Who is most at risk for school removal? A multilevel discrete-time survival analysis of individual- and context-level influences. *Journal of Educational Psychology* 103:223–237.

Pianta, R. C., W. S. Barnett, M. Burchinal, and K. R. Thornburg. 2009. The effects of preschool education: What we know, how public policy is or is not aligned with the evidence base, and what we need to know. *Psychological Science in the Public Interest* 10:49–88.

Raffaele-Mendez, L. M. 2003. Predictors of suspension and negative school outcomes: A longitudinal investigation. *New Directions for Youth Development* 99:17–33.

Reynolds, A. J., J. A. Temple, B. A. White, S. R. Ou, and D. L. Robertson. 2011. Age 26 cost-benefit analysis of the child-parent center early education program. *Child Development* 82:379–404.

Schweinhart, L. J., J. Montie, Z. Xiang, W. S. Barnett, C. R. Belfield, and M. Nores. 2005. *Lifetime effects: The High/Scope Perry Preschool Study through age 40.* Ypsilanti, MI: High/Scope Press. Pp. 194–215.

Skiba, R. J., R. S. Michael, A. C. Nardo, and R. L. Peterson. 2002. The color of discipline: Sources of racial and gender disproportionality in school punishment. *Urban Review* 34:317–342.

Skiba, R. J., R. H. Horner, C. G. Chung, M. Rausch, S. L. May, and T. Tobin, 2011. Race is not neutral: A national investigation of African American and Latino disproportionality in school discipline. *School Psychology Review* 40:85–107.

Standing together against suspension and expulsion in early childhood: A joint statement. 2016. Available from http://www.naeyc.org/files/naeyc/Standing%20Together.Joint%20Statement.FINAL_.pdf.

St. John, M. S., K. Thomas, and C. R. Noroña. 2012. Infant mental health professional development: Together in the struggle for social justice. *Zero to Three* 33(2):13–22.

Todd, A. R., K. C. Thiem, and R. Neel. 2016. Does seeing faces of young black boys facilitate the identification of threatening stimuli? *Psychological Science* 27:384–393.

Van Egeren, L. A., R. Kirk, H. E. Brophy-Herb, J. S. Carlson, B. Tableman, and S. Bender. 2011. *An interdisciplinary evaluation report of Michigan's Child Care Expulsion Prevention (CCEP) initiative.* East Lansing, MI: Michigan State University.

van Nunspeet, F., N. Ellemers, and B. Derks. 2015. Reducing implicit bias: How moral motivation helps people refrain from making "automatic" prejudiced associations. *Translational Issues in Psychological Science* 1:382–391.

Whitebook, M., C. McLean, and L. J. E. Austin. 2016. *Early childhood workforce index—2016.* Berkeley, CA: Center for the Study of Child Care Employment, University of California, Berkeley.

White House. 2014. *My Brother's Keeper Task Force report to the President.* Available from https://www.whitehouse.gov/sites/default/files/docs/053014_mbk_report.pdf.

White House Council of Economic Advisors. 2014. *The economics of early childhood investments.* Available from https://www.whitehouse.gov/sites/default/files/docs/the_economics_of_early_childhood_investments.pdf.

7

LESSONS FOR HEALTH EQUITY: MILITARY MEDICINE AS A WINDOW TO UNIVERSAL HEALTH INSURANCE

Jeff Hutchinson, MD, FAAP, Raquel Mack, MS, Tracey Pérez Koehlmoos, PhD, MHA, and Patrick H. DeLeon, PhD, MPH, JD

Health disparities result from multifaceted variables including access to health care and discrimination associated with socioeconomic status, education, social support, insurance, race, ethnicity, and gender. The purpose of this paper is to identify lessons learned and future research opportunities from the two national health systems that model universal health care: the Military Health System (MHS) and the Department of Veterans Affairs (VA). The concept that insurance and access are the primary factors in health disparities is partially supported in the MHS, yet mental health care remains disparate especially in posttraumatic stress disorder treatment and outcomes in the VA system. The data available from the VA and MHS demonstrate both elimination of disparities and areas where disparities continue despite equal access and resources. Increased focus on these health care delivery systems has the potential to clarify sources and solutions to health disparities.

DIVERSE DEMOGRAPHICS OF MILITARY MEMBERS, THEIR FAMILIES, AND PROVIDERS

The most recent demographics report over 3.6 million military personnel which include Department of Defense (DoD) active duty military personnel (1,326,273), active duty Coast Guard (39,454), DoD Ready Reserve and Coast Guard Reserve members (1,101,939), the Retired Reserve (214,784) and Standby Reserve (13,700), and DoD civilian personnel (856,484) (DoD, 2014). The following total military force demographics represent the 2.5 million members who are active duty and Selected Reserve. The Army accounts for 47 percent of the total military force. The Air Force, Navy, and Marine

Corps constitute 21, 17, and 12 percent, respectively, with the remaining 2 percent members of the Coast Guard. The total military force is mostly male with 16.2 percent female. The majority are white (71.0 percent), followed by black (16.8 percent), Asian (3.8 percent), American Indian or Alaska Native (1.2 percent), and Native Hawaiian or Other Pacific Islander (0.9 percent). The 2013 demographic report identifies 2.4 percent of the military members as multiracial, with 11 percent identified as having Hispanic ethnicity. The majority of the total military force is married (51 percent), and the largest age group is 25 years or younger (40 percent). There are more family members (2.98 million) than active duty and Selected Reserve (2.20 million) members. Active duty members' children are mostly between birth and 5 years (42 percent), followed by 6 to 11 years (31 percent), then 12 to 18 years (22 percent), and finally 19 to 22 years (4 percent).

There were 9.53 million beneficiaries eligible for DoD medical care including TRICARE Reserve Select, TRICARE Young Adult, and TRICARE Retired Reserve in 2014 (DHA DHCAPE, 2014). Providers who care for military members and their families are required to maintain the national standards for credentialing and certification in all military treatment facilities (MTFs) and civilian facilities where care is purchased. The quality of care in MTFs is held to the same national benchmarks as in civilian organizations. There are no copayments in the VA or MHS, and procedure and treatment approvals are based on medical justification. The use of an electronic medical record that can share information across the United States and internationally distinguishes care in and out of military facilities and the VA. The racial, gender, and ethnic background of providers in these systems should mirror the national provider demographics. Uniformed providers embody the additional diversity of experience and geographic relocation associated with the mobility of service. Awareness of military service and a positive bias toward military members and their families is a common thread for providers in these systems.

TWO DISTINCT SYSTEMS OF MILITARY HEALTH CARE

Although frequently confused by nonmilitary personnel, the MHS is separate from the VA health services. MHS primarily serves the active duty population, their family members as well as some retirees, whereas the VA exclusively treats veterans, a generally older cohort. The VA system is part of the Department of Veterans Affairs, and MHS is overseen by DoD. Not all veterans receive their health care through the VA system, and many who are of working age and in good health opt for private health insurance through their employer.

The Senate Appropriations Committee estimates that the Department of Veterans Affairs is responsible for providing care to approximately 48.3 million Americans, or 15 percent of the nation's population. The VA has the nation's largest integrated health care system, consisting of 167 medical centers, 1,018 community-based outpatient clinics, 300 Vet centers, and 135 community-based living centers.

The mission of the VA is to fulfill President Lincoln's promise, "To care for him who shall have borne the battle, and for his widow, and his orphan," by serving and honoring the men and women who are America's veterans. According to its mission statement:

America's Military Health System (MHS) is a unique partnership of medical educators, medical researchers, and health care providers and their support personnel worldwide. It is prepared to respond anytime, anywhere with comprehensive medical capability to military operations, natural disasters and humanitarian crises around the globe, and to ensure delivery of world-class health care to all DoD service members, retirees, and their families. The MHS promotes a fit, healthy and protected force by reducing non-combat losses, optimizing healthy behavior and physical performance, and providing casualty care. (Office of the Under Secretary for Personnel and Readiness, Health Affairs Mission)

The differences in health outcomes are influenced by the different patient populations, organizational structure, and priority. The similarities in decreased disparities are most likely the result of electronic medical record use, similar provider cohorts, and a single insurer.

CHALLENGES OF THE VA HEALTH CARE MISSION

A veteran is defined as anyone who has served in the Armed Forces. The current veteran population is approximately 21 million and expected to decrease to approximately 14 million by the year 2040, while the percentage of minority and female veterans is expected to increase (NCVAS, 2014). The black veteran population is expected to experience the greatest increase, from 12 to 16 percent, followed by the Hispanic veteran population growing from 7 to 11 percent; other races are expected to grow from 4 to 6 percent by the year 2040 (NCVAS, 2014). Health benefits in either the VA or MTF are prioritized to those who retire from active duty service and those with conditions related to service. Priority at VA facilities goes to veterans with an illness possibly related to their service in combat operations identified within 5 years after discharge and those with greater than 50 percent disability. There is no enrollment fee, monthly premium, or deductibles, and out-of-pocket costs are low or nonexistent (VA, 2015). There are several performance measure topics of interest for the Veterans Health Administration (VHA), including quality, timely access, patient-centered satisfaction and function, equitable community health, and efficient cost-effectiveness (Perlin et al., 2004). Although the VHA has made great strides to improve its services, there are still barriers to health care for veterans, including availability to rural populations and individual perceptions of the quality of care that affect the utilization of services. The distance to services and provider shortage in rural areas have been previously identified as barriers for veterans seeking health care within the VA system, specifically for common diagnostic services, routine specialty care, and emergency services.

HEALTH DISPARITIES FOR SERVICE MEMBERS AND VETERANS

Center for Health Equity Research and Promotion investigators have published over 445 scientific manuscripts in peer-reviewed journals, including at least 241 related to research on improving health quality and equity and care for vulnerable veteran populations since 2009. Mental health care is a known disparity. Military personnel have a high risk of developing psychological problems, especially when exposed to combat, and mental health services are not used by all personnel (Kehle et al., 2010; Ryan et al., 2007). Fewer than half experiencing mental health problems are likely to seek professional mental health care for fear of stigma or other related barriers to care (Ouimette et al., 2011). For example, there is an underuse of mental health care services among Operation Enduring Freedom/Operation Iraqi Freedom personnel, although there is a high prevalence of posttraumatic stress disorder (PTSD) within this population (Vogt, 2011). In 2011, Dawne Vogt conducted a review on empirical articles about mental health beliefs in military and veteran populations and found concerns about public stigma and personal mental health–related beliefs that may serve as important barriers to mental health care use (Murdoch et al., 2003). Military members and veterans have been categorized as underutilizers of mental health services, thought primarily to stem from cultural influences and a pervasive stigma associated with the appearance of being "weak." African American veterans have been far less likely than Caucasian veterans and those of other racial and/or ethnic groups to be classified as PTSD in order to receive medical treatment for a service-connected disorder (Harris, 2011; Nayback, 2008). Similar disparate care in the treatment of African American veterans for cardiac care, laparoscopic cholecystectomy, and carotid artery imaging has also been shown (Conigliaro et al., 2000; Harris, 2011).

ACCESS TO HEALTH CARE ELIMINATES SOME DISPARITY

Traditional definitions of disparities include those differences in outcomes that persist when access is equal. The Institute of Medicine study *Unequal Treatment* defined disparities as racial or ethnic differences in health care that were not due to access-related factors or clinical needs, preferences, and appropriateness of intervention (IOM, 2003). Thus, we would expect to see a lack of disparities in the military health care system because it provides universal coverage for all active duty service members, their families, many retirees, and the families of deceased service members. A recent example demonstrating the lack of disparities includes a rigorous look at emergency general surgery (EGS) outcomes over a 5-year period. The study found that risk-adjusted survival analyses found a lack of significant mortality and readmission differences at 30, 90, and 180 days. Although overall morbidity was higher among black versus white patients (HR [95% CI]—30-day HR = 1.23[1.13-1.35], 90-day HR = 1.18 [1.09-1.28], 180-day HR = 1.15 [1.07-1.24]) this finding seemingly was driven by appendiceal disorders (HR = 1.69-1.70) (Zogg et al., 2015). This lack of disparities in EGS is a situation not reflected in the general U.S. population. Thus, as many minority patients are also uninsured, increasing access to care such as through universal coverage like the MHS is thought to be a viable solution to mitigate inequities.

Ongoing research by the Comparative Effectiveness and Provider Induced Demand Collaboration team at the Uniformed Services University of the Health Sciences and Brigham & Women's Hospital indicates a lack of disparities across a variety of health- and surgery-related access and outcomes including maternal, cancer, and heart surgery procedures. Where racial disparities may be eliminated or insignificant, caution must be taken to search for rank-related disparities that may be unique to the military culture or may be more reliant on health literacy and training.

ADDRESSING BIAS MAY FURTHER DECREASE HEALTH DISPARITIES

Recent evidence of a lack of racial disparities in MHS may reflect the military value of "taking care of our own," which can serve as a unique equalizer among active duty patients and providers in this closed, universal coverage system.

Provider variability and geographic variation likely impact health care disparities after eliminating the variables of insurance and access to care. Cultural factors of disparities arise from gender, religion, race, ethnicity, and any shared group experience (Harris, 2011). Race-based cultural distrust of military medicine is not eliminated immediately upon entering the service. Howard Ross has stated that "Bias is like breathing" to emphasize that everyone has bias (Ross, 2014). Several biases remain in place even after universal coverage eliminates access and resource discrepancies.

The "bandwagon effect" happens when our decisions are influenced by a larger group's decision (Croskerry, 2003). Military medicine is particularly prone to this bias with a culture founded on discipline and standardization. Sick call was once organized by having every sick person report early in the morning between 5:00 and 6:00 AM, for providers to quickly identify those who were "really" sick. The low compassion and the belief that the majority were trying to miss duty contributed to errors in triage by both nonmedical supervisors and medical personnel and the eventual elimination of the system. Family members may also experience a bandwagon effect when providers see encounters as patients abusing a system that they consider free. For example, during a deployment, children are brought in to be seen more frequently (Gorman et al., 2010) which may negatively influence provider compassion. The transition to the medical home model for beneficiaries may reduce this effect as providers develop continuity with their patients.

Another bias is the clustering illusion, which happens when we see groupings, streaks, or clusters of a condition and apply the condition to a group (Croskerry, 2003). New military recruits, officers, different branches of the service, and units with unique reputations are often seen as homogeneous. When several patients present with a sexually transmitted infection, the racial assumptions apply but also the assumptions associated with their military designation. The military medical system adds another potential categorization to patients that may be grouped together.

Health care providers in a system with universal coverage no longer have the heuristic of poor health caused strictly by being poor without access to health care and may look to personality or behavioral traits to attribute a condition.

FUTURE RESEARCH OR POLICIES

The federal health care system provides an excellent vehicle for objectively exploring the underlying determinants of health disparities. Factors that have been explored in other settings may be verified as dependent upon access.

Other areas that continue to demonstrate disparity require exploration of new variables that contribute to health disparities such as rank and service to improve military and veteran health care. Theoretically, the traditional barriers of access, patient and provider economic concerns, and provider shortages should explain disparate outcomes. When differences remain, other sources require investigation. The expansion of telehealth within the DoD and VA to provide care and virtual advanced specialty care is another potential area in which to evaluate disparate outcomes in similar settings. The more subtle, and therefore traditionally less studied, cultural, social, and emotional factors may be playing a more critical role than appreciated. Future exploration is needed of the extent that different subpopulations possess differential health literacy capabilities as well as the influence of patient and provider preconceived expectations and the effects of an illness-oriented system versus a wellness-oriented system. Can universal care shift the focus from treating disease to preventive medicine and healthy lifestyle factors such as sleep, exercise, nutrition, and systematic stress reduction?

SUMMARY OF LESSONS LEARNED

The health disparities assumed to relate to a socioeconomic system that is separate and unequal should resolve in a universal health system like the MHS and VA. Some evidence exists that mandated care such as dental care for service members does eliminate disparities, but other areas remain. The delivery of the care contributes to the quality of the care, such as sick call versus a medical home. Lastly, culture exists outside of the military system and the culture from the military system is more likely to mix with instead of replace the effects of society outside of the military. Treatment and outcome improvement should be seen when care is both available and mandated yet the discrepancies that remain in a universal health system highlight the impact of culture, bias, and a focus on illness rather than wellness and prevention.

REFERENCES

Conigliaro, J., J. Whittle, C. B. Good, B. H. Hanusa, L. J. Passman, R. P. Lofgren, R. Allman, P. A. Ubel, M, O'Connor, and D. S. Macpherson. 2000. Understanding racial variation in the use of coronary revascularization procedures: The role of clinical factors. *Archives of Internal Medicine* 160(9):1329–1335.
Croskerry, P. 2003. The importance of cognitive errors in diagnosis and strategies to minimize them. *Academic Medicine* 78(8):775–780.

DHA DHCAPE (Defense Health Agency, Defense Health Cost Assessment and Program Evaluation). 2014. *Evaluation of the TRICARE program: access, cost, and quality, fiscal year 2014 report to Congress.* Available from http://health.mil/Military-Health-Topics/Access-Cost-Quality-and-Safety/Health-Care-Program-Evaluation/Annual-Evaluation-of-the-TRICARE-Program (accessed January 13, 2015).

DoD (Department of Defense). 2014. *2014 Demographics: Profile of the military community.* Available from http://download.militaryonesource.mil/12038/MOS/Reports/2014-Demographics-Report.pdf (accessed January 11, 2015).

Gorman, G. H., M. Eide, and E. Hisle-Gorman. 2010. Wartime military deployment and increased pediatric mental and behavioral health complaints. *Pediatrics* 126(6): 1058–1066.

Harris, G. L. 2011. Reducing healthcare disparities in the military through cultural competence. *Journal of Health & Human Services Administration* 34(2):145–181.

IOM (Institute of Medicine). 2003. *Unequal treatment: Confronting racial and ethnic disparities in health care,* edited by B. Smedley, A. Stith, and A. Nelson. Washington, DC: The National Academies Press.

Kehle, S. M., M. A. Polusny, M. Murdoch, C. R. Erbes, P. A. Arbisi, P. Thuras, and L. A. Meis. 2010. Early mental health treatment-seeking among U.S. National Guard soldiers deployed to Iraq. *Journal of Traumatic Stress* 23(1):33–40.

Murdoch, M., J. Hodges, C. Hunt, D. Cowper, N. Kressin, and N. O'Brien. 2003. Gender differences in service connection for PTSD. *Medical Care* 41(8):950–961.

Nayback, A. M. 2008. Health disparities in military veterans with PTSD: Influential sociocultural factors. *Journal of Psychosocial Nursing* 46(6):41–51.

NCVAS (National Center for Veterans Analysis and Statistics). 2014. *Projected veteran population 2013 to 2043.* Available from www.va.gov/vetdata/docs/quickfacts/population_slideshow.pdf.

Office of the Under Secretary for Personnel and Readiness. Health Affairs Mission. Available from http://prhome.defense.gov/HA/Mission (accessed October 18, 2016).

Ouimette, P., D. Vogt, M. Wade, V. Tirone, M. A. Greenbaum, R. Kimerling, C. Laffaye, J. E. Fitt, and C. S. Rosen. 2011. Perceived barriers to care among Veterans Health Administration patients with posttraumatic stress disorder. *Psychological Services* 8(3):212–223.

Perlin, J. B., R. M. Kolodner, and R. H. Roswell. 2004. The Veterans Health Administration: Quality, value, accountability, and information as transforming strategies for patient-centered care. *American Journal of Managed Care* 10(11 Pt 2):828–836.

Ross, H. 2014. *Everyday bias: Identifying and navigating unconscious judgments in our daily lives.* Rowman & Littlefield Publishers.

Ryan, M. A., T. C. Smith, B. Smith, P. Amoroso, E. J. Boyko, G. C. Gray, G. D. Gackstetter, J. R. Riddle, T. S. Wells, G. Gumbs, T. E. Corbeil, and T. I. Hooper. 2007. Millennium cohort: Enrollment begins a 21-year contribution to understanding the impact of military service. *Journal of Clinical Epidemiology* 60(2):181–191.

VA (U.S. Department of Veterans Affairs). 2015. *Health benefits.* Available from http://www.va.gov/healthbenefits/apply/returning_servicemembers.asp.

Vogt, D. 2011. Mental health-related beliefs as a barrier to service use for military personnel and veterans: A review. *Psychiatric Services* 62(2):135–142.

Zogg, C. K., W. Jiang, M. A. Chaudhary, A. A. Shah, S. R. Lipsitz, J. S. Weissman, Z. Cooper, A. Salim, S. L. Nitzchke, L. L. Nguyen, L. A. Helmchen, L. Kimsey, S. T. Olaiya, P. A. Learn, and A. H. Haider. 2015. *Racial disparities in emergency general surgery: Do difference in outcomes persist in universally-insured military patients?* Paper presented at the 74th Annual Meeting of the American Association for the Surgery of Trauma and Clinical Congress of Acute Care Surgery, Las Vegas, NV.

8

PRINCIPLES OF ADOLESCENT- AND YOUNG-ADULT-FRIENDLY CARE: CONTRIBUTIONS TO REDUCING HEALTH DISPARITIES AND INCREASING HEALTH EQUITY

Angela Diaz, MD, PhD, MPH, and Ken Peake, DSW

Adolescents (ages 10 to 19) and young adults (ages 20 to 24) make up approximately 21 percent of the population of the United States (U.S. Census Bureau, 2016). Adolescents are widely considered to be a population at the crossroads of lifelong good or poor health because adolescence is a time characterized by experimentation fueled by the drive for independence. Experimentation for many adolescents includes behaviors that may involve risk exposure that can impact long-term health and well-being. But, young adulthood, though relatively overlooked, is an equally critical developmental period, in which young people are expected to take on new responsibilities and to begin to establish themselves in the world (IOM and NRC, 2014). Behavioral patterns, lifestyles, and health-service-utilization patterns evolve during this stage of life to mold health over the life course.

Health care providers can play a unique role in providing appropriate interventions that encourage young people to become good health care consumers and adopt healthy behaviors. These interventions can be reinforced by educators, advocates, and families to empower young people to thrive physically and emotionally. Yet, despite young people's deep potential to contribute to our society if they are given the opportunity for a healthy present and future, their unique needs are not adequately addressed by either pediatric or adult-focused health care models. For both adolescents and young adults, lack of health care and health risk behaviors can result in health disparities further down the road and increase the risk for developing chronic diseases later in life. Disturbingly, by young adulthood, we find a magnification of health disparities that interfere with a successful transition to adulthood (IOM and NRC, 2014).

We argue that providing health services that are adolescent and young-adult friendly (i.e., specifically designed to account for the characteristics of young people) can improve both their access to and utilization of health care. Therefore, this paper outlines the key principles that we propose should guide the design and delivery of adolescent and young-adult care.

HEALTH DISPARITIES IN THE ADOLESCENT AND YOUNG-ADULT POPULATIONS

While the causes of health disparities are highly complex and still too poorly understood, certain social factors are known to be associated with these disparities in the adolescent and young-adult populations. For instance, poverty has long been associated with health disparities among young people. Adolescents who are poor report worse health outcomes, including higher rates of sexually transmitted infections and pregnancy, than higher-socioeconomic-status (SES) adolescents (Gold et al., 2002). They also have higher rates of depression and suicide and are more likely to be sexually abused or victims of homicide (Fiscella and Williams, 2004). Obesity is also higher among low-SES adolescents than those who are better off (Miech et al., 2006).

Young adults, who are often thought to be a naturally robust population when compared to older people, face declining health and challenges related to mental health, wellness, and obesity. These factors, among others, are inherently linked to their long-term health (IOM and NRC, 2014). Similar to adolescents, low-SES young adults have poorer health outcomes than those who are better off (Hudson et al., 2013; Mulye et al., 2009).

Geography

Where adolescents and young adults live also has an impact on health disparities; young people who live in rural areas are more likely to be poor and less educated than those who live in or near urban and suburban environments, and both factors are associated with a range of poorer health outcomes (HHS, 2016; USDA, 2015). Young people from rural areas commonly have less access to primary health care and mental health care (Rural Health Association, 2016).

Race/Ethnicity

Adolescents and young adults of color face health disparities associated with their race and ethnicity (IOM and NRC, 2014). Those who are African American, American Indian or Alaska Native, or Latino experience worse outcomes in a variety of areas compared to adolescents who are white (Elster et al., 2003; Hudson et al., 2013; Neumark-Sztainer et al., 2002; Singh et al., 2008; Vo and Park, 2008). When compared to whites, African American and Latino fifth-graders have higher rates of exposure to violence, peer victimization, substance use, and terrorism worries; lower rates of seat-belt use, bike-helmet use, and vigorous exercise; and lower self-rated health status and psychological and physical quality of life (Schuster et al., 2012). These conditions mean that addressing racial and ethnic disparities will become even more pressing in the next decade if progress is to be made toward health equity. Also, the adolescent and young-adult populations are becoming more ethnically and racially diverse, with steady growth in the proportions of these age groups who are youth of color, particularly Latinos and Asian American youth.

Sexual Orientation

Among the youth population, lesbian, gay, bisexual, and transgender (LGBT) youth are particularly vulnerable to a range of health disparities. LGBT adolescents and young adults have significantly worse health outcomes than heterosexual youth, including higher rates of mental health problems, including chronic stress and depression, as well as suicide. These outcomes are significantly related to discrimination, harassment, and other forms of victimization, which takes place in families, schools, and communities (Burton et al., 2013; Saewyc, 2011).

HEALTH CARE ACCESS AND UTILIZATION

While we recognize that disparate health outcomes for young people involve complex interactions among multiple factors, a potentially protective factor that can change the health trajectory for young people is access to age-appropriate health care and utilization of services. Young people who experience multiple risk factors, already mentioned, may also lack health-insurance coverage and age-appropriate services. As a result, the current health care delivery system is not meeting the challenges young people face today; this means there are many missed opportunities (IOM and NRC, 2009, 2014).

The Affordable Care Act and the Future

How health disparities among adolescents and young adults will be influenced in the long term by any of the various initiatives for health-insurance reform, including the Affordable Care Act (ACA) or its potential replacements, remains unclear. More than 40 percent of those affected by coverage expansion under the ACA were poor, young people of color (National Conference of State Legislatures, 2011). In 2010, the first year after the implementation of the ACA, and in 2011, spending on young-adult health grew faster than for other age groups, but it appears that emergency-room use and psychiatric and substance-abuse hospitalizations may account for much of this growth in spending (Health Care Cost Institute, 2014). Access to primary care services for young adults has improved, but this age group is still the most likely to be uninsured (30 percent) compared to any other age group (Centers for Medicare & Medicaid Services, 2016).

Adolescents

Adolescents have long received less health care than all other age groups (Irwin et al., 2009; Newacheck et al., 2004), with the exception of young adults (IOM and NRC, 2014). But, although the ACA has significantly increased coverage for adolescents, there remain concerns about whether they will get all the care they need, even if it is to survive. Adolescents are known to forego care when they fear that their confidentiality and privacy might be compromised, and important remaining obstacles include a lack of awareness of eligible benefits under ACA, lack of youth confidentiality, and discomfort and stigma (Advocates for Youth, 2017). One problem is seen in the low rates of provision of long-acting reversible contraception (LARCs): "A lack of awareness of benefits, confidentiality concerns, and discomfort and stigma on the part of providers all play a role and contribute to low rates of use of LARCs in young people, even though this method is highly effective at preventing pregnancy and is cost effective over time" (Advocates for Youth, 2017).

Young Adults

The health of young adults has received inadequate attention, given that their health outcomes are even worse than those of adolescents. Indeed, despite the myth that young adults are healthy, young adulthood is a time when we see an alarming drop in a range of indicators of health and well-being (IOM and NRC, 2014). Even compared to adolescents, who have low rates of health care utilization compared to all other age groups, young adults have the lowest rates of health care utilization and significantly higher emergency-room use compared to both adolescents and adults (IOM and NRC, 2014). The ACA provided coverage for more than 3 million young adults who were added to health-insurance rolls in the first two years of implementation, which increased routine health care visits by this age group and greatly reduced levels of care foregone because of cost (Claxton et al., 2012). But, currently, with calls to dismantle the ACA and replace it, the future remains very unclear.

Unmet Needs

The marked disparities in health care use between adolescents and young adults and other age groups have been attributed to the idea that these age groups have fewer needs. It is a myth that young people do not need services. In fact, they have significant unmet health needs (Ames, 2008). Among adolescents, 9 percent of all 10- to 17-year olds and 12 percent of poor 10- to 17-year olds have limitation of activity due to a chronic health condition (McManus and Fox, 2007). Even for adolescents and young adults who are generally in good health, access to health care, preventive care, and health education is necessary to ensure continued good health throughout their lives (National Conference of State Legislatures 2011).

Unaddressed mental health problems, while disturbingly high among adolescents, are of even greater concern in young adults. Only 20 percent of adolescents with serious mental health conditions get proper care, but by young adulthood, this rate is cut in half. Only 10 percent of young adults with serious mental health conditions get care (Fox et al., 2010b).

Disparities in Health Care Access

There are longstanding disparities in access to and use of health care among adolescents. For example, in a 2003 study conducted after Medicaid expansion and the creation of State Children's Health Insurance Programs, low-SES adolescents remained at a significant disadvantage, with less access to care and less health care utilization when compared to middle-class adolescents (Irwin et al., 2009). Young adults, who historically have had lower rates of insurance than children and adolescents, have even less access and utilization. For many, and particularly among vulnerable groups such as youth of color and LGBT youth, the situation is more dire (IOM and NRC, 2014; National Conference of State Legislatures, 2011; Vo and Park, 2008).

Even with implementation of the ACA, the estimated share of youth ages 10–19 who are eligible but uninsured varies from 2.3 percent in Massachusetts to 17.8 percent in Texas (Office of Disease Prevention and Health Promotion, 2016). Since the ACA, many low-income older adolescents (particularly those ages 19 and 20) remain uninsured in 22 states where there are no subsidies provided to them or where Medicaid has not been expanded. This is particularly important as this group is unlikely to have employer-based coverage or coverage under a parent's private insurance plan (Fox et al., 2013b).

MEETING THE HEALTH CARE NEEDS OF ADOLESCENTS AND YOUNG ADULTS

Reducing health disparities that result from lack of care involves far more than ensuring that young people have insurance coverage or can find and reach services. Both adolescents and young adults have population-specific characteristics and concerns that must be taken into account if they are to make use of services. Young people may forego care or avoid talking about vital issues with a health care provider if services are insensitive to their needs and providers are uncomfortable with or unprepared to address their issues (Lehrer et al., 2007).

Despite this, the current care-transformation activities under the ACA and Primary Care Medical Home (PCMH) initiatives, have not taken into account the unique needs of adolescents and young adults (Stille et al., 2010; Walker et al., 2011). The PCMH, which originated as a way to improve quality of care through a partnership between the patient or family and a highly coordinated and comprehensive network of providers (Sia et al., 2004), is defined by the Agency for Healthcare Research and Quality (AHRQ) as a model for the improvement of primary care nationally that emphasizes core functions such as: comprehensiveness (with care provided by a multidisciplinary team); patient-centered (with patients as fully informed partners in care planning, with understanding and respect of each patient's unique needs, culture, values, and preferences); a high level of coordination; accessibility; and a commitment to quality and quality improvement (AHRQ, 2017). Because this transformation effort originated from a chronic-care model focused initially on the health care needs of the elderly and children with special needs in an effort to create cost savings for populations with high care utilization, the needs of adolescents and young adults have not been given adequate consideration (Fox et al., 2013a).

Therefore, it should not be a surprise that, while the American Academy of Pediatrics framework for the PCMH recommends that "developmentally appropriate and culturally competent health assessments and counseling" be used to "ensure successful transition to adult-oriented health care, work, and independence" (American Academy of Pediatrics, 2016), there are no specific recommendations with regard to adolescents and their concerns about privacy, confidentiality, and stigma. One of the aims of this paper is to describe the unique characteristics of young people that should be considered in designing their health services.

Giving due consideration to these unique concerns and issues when delivering health services for them is what we mean by the term "adolescent- and young-adult-friendly approach." This approach is intended to ensure that services are easily accessible, meet the needs of young people (particularly the most vulnerable), and are designed in a way that makes them acceptable to young people (i.e., young people will use them comfortably and responsibly). Acceptability and appropriateness are known to influence the willingness of young people to use services (Resnick et al., 1980). To achieve this end, we argue that the multiple barriers to care must be met to ensure appropriate service design and delivery for this population. We highlight several of these barriers below.

Confidentiality

A major potential barrier to seeking care for adolescents is their concern about confidentiality and the fact that they will commonly avoid services if they feel their privacy is in danger of being violated (Lehrer et al., 2007). While many states have confidentiality laws on the books with regard to adolescents, providers are generally uninformed about the rights of adolescents to confidential services (Huppert and Adams Hillard, 2003; Reddy et al., 2002). In our experience, young adults, despite not being minors, have similar concerns to adolescents about privacy and frequently do not want a parent to know about their health care visit. While ACA's extension of insurance coverage under a parent's plan until age 26 years has led to increased insurance coverage for young adults, the explanation of benefits (EOB) that private insurance companies send to the policyholder creates a problem that may deter many from seeking care for privacy-sensitive services.

Service Provider Relationship

Adolescents are more likely to place importance on the personal characteristics of their medical provider than are adults, and they report that health care providers do not spend enough time to get to know them and focus on their problems rather than on their strengths (Fox et al., 2010b). The Positive Youth Development (PYD) framework (Larson, 2000; Pittman et al., 2000), embraced by the Mount Sinai Adolescent Health Center (MSAHC) (Diaz et al., 2005), is a widely accepted guide to the design of services for young people to ensure that they are acceptable and well utilized by young people. PYD offers a framework that takes into consideration the contribution of social and institutional factors (including protective factors) to adolescent resilience and vulnerability. PYD focuses on the fit between the opportunities for meaningful participation that are necessary for healthy development and the characteristics of the communities and institutions within which young people live. It starts with the maxim that for a young person to be "problem-free is not [to be] fully prepared" for the future (Pittman et al., 2000, p. 20), as problems and challenges are instrumental to developing an individual's personal and social assets (Scales and Leffert, 1999). These assets include motivation to develop new skills; self-efficacy and sense of responsibility for self; critical thinking; emotional self-regulation; good relationships with peers, parents, or other adults; and a sense of having good health-risk-management skills. Key to development of these assets is the role of adults in finding ways to be able to allow adolescents gradual and increasing control over personal decision making while remaining available for guidance when it is sought (Eccles et al., 1993; Larson, 2000). For a description of PYD in health care delivery, see Diaz et al. (2005).

Unfortunately, most health-services providers may not know about the concerns that young people have when seeking care: young people report that they are infrequently asked to give any feedback regarding the health services they receive (Fox et al., 2013). Although much of the knowledge about issues in serving young people has come from studies conducted among adolescents and has been insufficiently studied in young adults, it is highly likely that the lessons learned from adolescents also largely apply—at least in broad strokes—to young adults. The experience gained in our health center, where we work with young people ages 10 through 24 years, suggests that young adults have many of the same concerns and experiences in seeking health care that they had as adolescents.

Even more disturbing than the fact that health-services providers who serve young people fail to get their feedback about how to best serve them is the fact that young people frequently report that their health providers fail to ask about sensitive issues, including sex and sexuality, substance abuse and other risky behaviors, as well as abuse and violence and other traumatic exposures, all of which are often at the core of adolescents' and young adults' experiences and concerns (Alexander et al., 2014; Klein and Wilson, 2002; Schoen et al., 1997).

Stigma

Both adolescents and young adults have concerns about being stigmatized or feeling shame and are extremely sensitive to the perceptions of others, including their peers (Woods and Neinstein, 2002). Therefore, the way that services are organized (whether under one roof or via a referral process) should be done in a way that is stigma free. For example, the way services are named can contribute to stigma: using terms such as "HIV services," " sexual assault services," "mental health services," and "family planning services" creates a stigma barrier. Furthermore, the way services are scheduled can inadvertently contribute to stigma if it is evident to others in the waiting room which service a young person is getting. For example, if "HIV services" are all scheduled in one clinic session, with few other services being provided at that time, for a young person simply being in the waiting room may lead to a fear of being exposed as HIV positive. This can present major challenges to small practices, but sensitivity to the issues of privacy and stigma is still a necessary consideration if young people are to feel comfortable and welcome.

Provider Preparation and Training

Health care providers in general often do not feel sufficiently prepared for or adept at dealing with the issues of young people. Many are not well trained to work with adolescents (Fox et al., 2010a), and a review of the literature suggests there has been insufficient attention given to the particular skills and knowledge that would prepare providers to work with young adults. Clinician-related barriers to adolescent care include provider insensitivity, lack of knowledge and skills regarding sexual and reproductive health, insufficient/inadequate communication, and discomfort with young people and their concerns and behaviors (Blum and Bearlinger, 1990; Blum et al., 1996), which can lead to young people feeling judged (Schuster et al., 1996). It is not clear that providers are any better prepared to address the health concerns and problems of young adults.

ADOLESCENT- AND YOUNG-ADULT-FRIENDLY SERVICES

Adolescent- and young-adult-friendly health services have at their foundation principles and heuristics for the design and delivery of care that have emerged from the field of adolescent and young-adult health over a four- or five-decade period. This approach evolved from the field of adolescent medicine in recognition of the unique developmental characteristics, concerns, vulnerabilities, and opportunities for health promotion of adolescents along with their relative inexperience in seeking or navigating health care independently. Because much of the work to date stems from work with adolescents and those transitioning to young adulthood, the full consideration of the needs and characteristic concerns of young adults is, in our view, a much-less-developed area, which presents an opportunity for us to learn much more. Despite this shortcoming, there is an emerging but still "loose" consensus about what should guide the design and delivery of health services for young people.

The Mount Sinai Adolescent Health Center: A Case Study

The Mount Sinai Adolescent Health Center (MSAHC), New York City, was given mention in the 2009 Institute of Medicine report *Adolescent Health Services: Missing Opportunities* (IOM and NRC, 2009) for its focus on a youth-development approach to health and as "noteworthy for its emphasis on youth empowerment through intentional engagement with adolescents and partners in understanding and ownership of their health" (p. 230). Furthermore, MSAHC's social-justice framework and its service principles have recently been articulated through a study being conducted by a team of researchers at ICF International, funded by the New York State Health Foundation, for the development of a Blueprint for

Adolescent and Young Adult Health Services (Mount Sinai Adolescent Health Center, 2017). The ICF International Research Team, as part of a third-party evaluation, studied and iterated the principles for adolescent and young-adult service development and provision embedded in the MSAHC model and simultaneously conducted a review of the literature to identify additional service principles for adolescent service models and guidelines. Table 8-1 lists the principles that are foundational to the MSAHC approach and the support for these principles that can be found in the literature. For brevity, rather than reviewing all the principles, we will focus on a few key principles that MSAHC considers in ensuring that its services are equitable and also acceptable to its diverse population of young consumers.

TABLE 8-1 | Principles That Guide the Design and Delivery of Adolescent and Young-Adult Health Services and Sources in the Literature

Equitable	All young people, not just selected groups, are able to obtain the health services and that services do not discriminate against any sector of youth on grounds of gender, ethnicity, religion, disability, social status, sexual orientation, or any other reason. (3, 4, 5, 15)
Reach out to the most vulnerable of those who lack services	Implement case-management services, including transportation assistance, to youth with HIV, mental health issues and other conditions that may be barriers to accessing care; focus on youth most vulnerable to risky behavior and poor health; remove barriers to care
Accessible and easily navigated	Geographically and financially accessible, easily identifiable, and easy to access for services both by appointment and walk-in (1, 2, 3, 4, 5,7, 8, 11, 14, 15, 17)
Comprehensive	Deliver an essential package of services, including preventive services, health promotion, risk-reduction counseling and education, and all-inclusive services (as many services as possible in one place) (3, 4, 7, 8, 9, 12, 17)
Integrated	Integration of primary and behavioral health care services; screen and refer for sexual and reproductive health issues, substance use, and mental health concerns (1, 9, 12, 17)
Confidential and obtaining informed consent from young people themselves	Separate waiting room for youth; adopt adolescent- and young-adult-sensitive authorization and review processes; guarantee confidentiality and adolescent minors' rights to consent to sexual and reproductive health care; informational, social, psychological, and physical privacy, beyond traditional confidentiality (1, 2, 3, 4, 6, 7, 10, 12, 13, 16, 17, 18)
Developmentally tailored and appropriate	Age-appropriate approach and health education materials, adolescent- and young-adult-friendly providers (2, 5, 7, 8)
Relationship-based	Mentorship of youth by providers; importance of relationships with providers on youth development; providers who spend enough time with the youth (8, 21)
Supportive of one-on-one youth–provider interactions	Parents of adolescent minors should be asked to wait in the waiting room and be reassured that they will be invited back in to discuss any remaining issues; once provider is alone with the teen, establish ground rules for confidentiality (22)

Sensitive, trained, and reflective staff	Staff receive training and support regarding working with adolescents and young adults; services are effective because they are delivered by trained and motivated health care providers; care provided by adolescent specialists; adolescent health resources and mechanisms for providers, including subspecialty sources of care and reference materials; provider collaboration; efficient division of responsibility (care delivered by most appropriate providers); staff sensitivity (to young people); compensation for providers; build staff capacity to serve adolescent patients (3, 4, 7, 10, 13, 16)
Safe space and approach that is nonjudgmental and without stigma	Welcoming with visual teaching aids; youth-friendly environment that signals diversity and the competence of the service to listen to and help with any concern or question, no matter what (1, 2, 3, 10, 17, 19)
Respectful	Providers who take youth seriously, listen, do not scold them; providers support youth in making their own decisions; exams are done with maximum respect for youth's dignity (1, 3)
Culturally competent	Culturally appropriate health education materials, celebrating diversity (1, 2, 5, 6, 7)
Promoting parent–child communication	Parental involvement encouraged in the care of adolescent minors but not required; elicit input and feedback from young people and their families; when serving teens, invite the parent back into room to discuss visit with youth and provider once confidentiality ground rules are agreed on without parent in exam room (1, 3, 7, 10, 22)

SOURCES

NATIONAL AND INTERNATIONAL ORGANIZATIONS

1. Advocates for Youth: Best Practices for Youth-Friendly Clinical Services* http://www.advocatesforyouth.org/publications/publications-a-z/1347--best-practices-for-youth-friendly-clinical-services Presented as best practices for youth-friendly clinics.

2. American College of Obstetricians and Gynecologists: The Initial Reproductive Health Visit http://www.acog.org/Resources-And-Publications/Committee-Opinions/Committee-on-Adolescent-Health-Care/The-Initial-Reproductive-Health-Visit Presented as "youth-friendly" clinic characteristics.

3   Engender Health: Youth-Friendly Services: A Manual for Service Providers https://www.engenderhealth.org/files/pubs/gender/yfs/yfs.pdf Presented as "youth-friendly" clinic characteristics.

4   Family Health International: Family Health International and the United Nations Population Fund Egypt. (2008). Training Manual for the Providers of Youth Friendly Services http://www.fhi360.org/resource/training-manual-providers-youth-friendly-services Presented as "youth-friendly" services.

5. Healthy Teen Network: "Is Your Clinic Youth Friendly? Why, What, How, and What's Next" http://www.hhs.gov/ash/oah/oah-initiatives/teen_pregnancy/training/Assests/2014%20Conference/youthfriendlyclinic.pdf Recommends same principles as the World Health Organization (see below).

6. International Planned Parenthood Federation: Keys to Youth Friendly: Introducing the Series http://www.ippf.org/sites/default/files/keys_introduction.pdf Presented as "keys" to improving youth-friendly services.

7. National Adolescent Health Information Center at the University of California, San Francisco: http://nahic.ucsf.edu/downloads/Assuring_Hlth_Checklist.pdf National Adolescent Health Information Center. (1998). Assuring the Health of Adolescents in Managed Care. San Francisco, CA: University of California, San Francisco, National Adolescent Health Information Center. Presented as components of adolescent health care delivery and includes a substantial checklist for planning and evaluating adolescent health care services.

8. National Alliance to Advance Adolescent Health: Adolescents' Experiences and Views on Health Care http://www.thenationalalliance.org/pdfs/Report2.%20Adolescents'%20Experiences%20and%20 Views%20on%20Health%20Care.pdf Presented as adolescents' views on how their health care should be delivered.

9. National Alliance to Advance Adolescent Health: http://gottransition.org/resourceGet. cfm?id=206

10. National Alliance to Advance Adolescent Health: Under One Roof: Primary Care Models That Work for Adolescents http://www.thenationalalliance.org/pdfs/Report1.%20Under%20One%20Roof%20-%20Primary%20 Care%20Models.pdf Presented as an "approach" to an adolescent-centered health care program. *MSAHC was profiled, along with three other adolescent clinics, for this article.

11. National Council of Community Behavioral Care: Is Your Organization Trauma Informed? http://www.thenationalcouncil.org/wp-content/uploads/2012/11/Is-Your-Organization-Trauma-Informed.pdf Offers guidelines for organization self-assessment and adoption of trauma-informed care practices and strategies.

12. Institute of Medicine: National Research Council and Institute of Medicine. (2009). *Adolescent Health Services: Missing Opportunities.* Committee on Adolescent Health Services and Models of Care for Treatment, Prevention and Healthy Development, R. S. Lawrence, J. Appleton Gootman, and L.J. Sim, Editors. Board of Children, Youth and Families. Division of Behavioral and Social Sciences and Education. Washington, D.C.: The National Academies Press. Presented as goals and practices.

13. SAMHSA-HRSA Center for Integrated Health Solutions: Improving Health Through Trauma-Informed Care. July 28, 2015 Webinar.

14. Society for Adolescent Medicine: Morreale, M., Kapphahn, C., Elster, A., Juszczak, L., Klein, J. (2004). Access to healthcare for adolescents and young adults: Position paper of the Society for Adolescent Medicine. *Journal of Adolescent Health* 35:342–344. Presented as recommendations for improving care of adolescents.

15. World Health Organization: Making health services adolescent friendly: Developing national quality standards for adolescent-friendly health services. http://apps.who.int/iris/bitstr eam/10665/75217/1/9789241503594_eng.pdf Presented as framework for adolescent-friendly health services.

HEALTH DEPARTMENTS

16. New York City Department of Health and Mental Hygiene Young Men's Health Initiative (no year): Best Practices in Sexual and Reproductive Health Care for Adolescents. For health care providers in primary care, family medicine, pediatrics, adolescent health, family planning and obstetrics and gynecology. Presented as "how-to" for making clinics youth friendly.

17. Labor, N., Kaplan, D., Graff, K. (2006). Healthy Teens Initiative: Seven Steps to Comprehensive Sexual and Reproductive Health Care for Adolescents in New York City. New York: New York City Department of Health and Mental Hygiene. Presented as best practices for meeting the health care needs of adolescents.

JOURNAL ARTICLES

18. Britto M., Tivorsak T., Slap, G. (2010). Adolescents' needs for health care privacy. *Pediatrics* 126(6):1469–1476. Discusses the array of confidentiality needs of adolescents and how they can be addressed in a clinic environment.

19. Dick B., Ferguson J., Chandra-Mouli V., Brabin L., et al. A review of the evidence for interventions to increase young people's use of health services in developing countries. In Ross, D., Dick, B., J Ferguson (Eds.). *Preventing HIV/AIDS in young people: A systematic review of the evidence from developing countries.* Geneva, World Health Organization, 2006. Identified several characteristics of youth health services in programs that showed some evidence of effectiveness.

20. Mandel, L., Qazilbash, J. (2005). Youth voices as change agents: Moving beyond the medical model in school-based health center practice. *Journal of School Health* 75(7):239–242. Examines the impact of youth involvement in a youth clinic.

21. Sale, E., Bellamy, N., Springer, J. F., & Wang, M. Q. (2008). Quality of provider-participant relationships and enhancement of adolescent social skills. *Journal of Primary Prevention* 29(3):263–278. Demonstrates the positive effect of relationship building with youth by health care and other social services providers.

MSAHC's framework utilizes PYD principles to strengthen young people's access and use of high-quality health care specifically designed to address their health care needs, their concerns, and the unique sensitivities that they may have about seeking and using care (Diaz et al., 2005). MSAHC recognizes that, during adolescence, the responsibility to be healthy begins to shift from parents and caregivers to young people, making it critical to ensure that young people have access to health care, education, and the opportunity to develop the skills they need to be productive and make valuable societal contributions (McNeely and Blanchard, 2009). MSAHC's mission is to "break down economic and social barriers to health care and wellness for young people by providing vital services—high-quality, comprehensive, confidential, and free—for all who come to us . . . [because] physical health and emotional well-being in adolescence is the foundation of a productive and fulfilling adult life [and] every teenager and young adult has the right to proactive, inclusive, and compassionate health care that demonstrably improves their chances of preventing disease and dysfunction . . . [an approach that helps them] become informed health consumers who take responsibility for their own well-being, benefiting them and society long term" (Mount Sinai Adolescent Health Center, 2016).

MSAHC provides free health services to more than 10,000 vulnerable young people ages 10 to 24 each year, of whom 98 percent are low income and 95 percent are of color. The service evolved to particularly attract and welcome young people who lack alternatives—for instance, those who are uninsured and poor—however, care is provided to any young person who seeks it and it is free. Their levels of education and household situations are extremely diverse; some are in foster care, homelessness, sex trafficking, or are refugees, while others have better life circumstances. Regardless, the MSAHC aims to provide a safe, welcoming, nonjudgmental environment in which young people can access high-quality health care.

The MSAHC model (Diaz et al., 2005; Mount Sinai Adolescent Health Center, 2017) is comprehensive, interdisciplinary, and highly integrated, with all services provided under one roof. At the core are primary health care, sexual and reproductive health care, dental care, optical care, and mental and behavioral health care. Primary medical care is delivered by specialists in adolescent medicine who provide preventive medical services, health maintenance, acute care, management of chronic illnesses, and inpatient services. Each adolescent knows his or her own provider who serves as both primary care practitioner and case manager for all health care needs. Mental health care includes individual, group, and family psychotherapy; psychological testing; psychiatric services; diagnostic and psychopharmacological services; and specialized care for mentally ill, traumatized, and substance-abusing youth. MSAHC provides specialized services for rape, incest, sexual-abuse, and sexual-assault survivors; for youth with eating disorders; for HIV+ youth; for teen parents (and their children); for transgender youth; and for LGBTQ youth.

Principle: Equitable Care

If all young people could obtain health services that did not discriminate against any sector of youth on grounds of gender, race, ethnicity, religion, disability, social status, and sexual orientation but instead were proactively designed to embrace and celebrate these diverse groups, disparities resulting from lack of access to and under-use of care might be greatly reduced.

Principle: Safe Space

One purpose of the adolescent- and young-adult-friendly approach is to ensure that all young people have a "safe space" where they can air concerns and questions without stigma or adult judgment. Many young people have not yet developed health literacy and have no experience navigating the silos by which health care is organized (Brown et al., 2007; Gray et al., 2005; Manganello, 2009). Yet, developmentally young people must learn to seek and use care on their own. Furthermore, many do not wish to disclose their concerns to a parent or caregiver, especially in regard to deeply personal issues like sexual health, gender identity, or risky behaviors. For some, the drive to seek care is created by a health crisis such as a suspected pregnancy or a sexually transmitted infection. For others the impetus is to obtain contraceptive counseling and contraceptives, or for other types of guidance. Some may be sick or may need an annual physical for sports participation or working papers. But, often the reason for the visit may not be initially transparent.

For example, our research shows that many young people at MSAHC who are victims of sexual assault or abuse may feel that they are somehow culpable, fear being blamed by adults and others, or do not recognize that what they experienced was abuse (Surko et al., 2005). Thus, they may not spontaneously reveal a history of trauma or know they need help. Therefore, it is essential that our service and providers minimize the need for a young person to be fully informed and health literate about their health conditions, concerns, or psychosocial needs in order to receive the services they need.

Principle: Coordinated and Easily Navigated Care

Vulnerable young people require a tailored approach that is sensitive to their concerns before the outreach stage and, when they enter a service, require a highly coordinated and easily navigable approach once they cross the threshold. For the highly vulnerable, marginalized by poverty, racial, and ethnic prejudice, or for those who might harbor distrust of "mainstream" institutions, the prospect of finding a place to go for health care is even more challenging. Many of the most marginalized young people may already have been stigmatized or rejected—in their schools, communities, and even by their families. For example, many lesbian, gay, bisexual, and questioning youth, have faced stigma on a very personal level, transgender youth especially so (Brown et al., 2007; Saewyc, 2011). Adolescents and young adults with chronic conditions like HIV are very fearful that they will be further stigmatized or rejected (Harper et al., 2014). Ensuring that *adolescent and young-adult services reach out to the most vulnerable youth* is one way to bridge them into services.

Principle: Safe Space

Creating easily identifiable and welcoming services is one component that can send the message that young people are valued and important. This is a first step in making the clinical space emotionally and physically safe (Lim et al., 2012). Young people report that office spaces which are unappealing or have little adolescent- and young-adult-specific information are a barrier to care (Fox et al., 2013; Lim et al., 2012). Creating a welcoming safe space includes making sure its appearance and messaging (digital media, posters, artwork, and brochures) communicates diversity and compassion, and this signals to the newcomer that no issue or question is off limits. Letting them know in this way that any issue is welcomed and, consequently, that staff are comfortable handling their issues is the first step in giving them permission to talk.

Principle: Accessibility

Creating services that are accessible, with no barriers at reception, and are easily navigated (especially when, as at MSAHC, they are comprehensive, integrated, and housed in one place) minimizes the burden on the young person to diagnose their own problems and to understand exactly what they need and how to ask for it. For example, it is common at MSAHC for both adolescents and young adults who have had traumatic exposure (the large majority of the patient population) to come in frequently with urgent needs such as a pregnancy or a sexually transmitted infection. We view it as our service's responsibility to draw clear connections between the presenting issue and the "real," underlying need. The MSAHC approach assumes that young people are still learning how to navigate on their own and do not have the experience by which to name and label their concerns. So we ask about all aspects of each young person's life, including their strengths, hopes, and areas of struggle.

Principle: Engagement

Engagement, which is necessary to maintain young people in care over time, is further encouraged via sensitive yet holistic questioning by the provider (Peake et al., 2005). This use of "active questioning" in inquiring about all aspects of a young person's life—including each person's hopes and aspirations—is an essential element in ensuring that the services they get span wellness, prevention, risk reduction, and treatment. The model of services put in place to support this continuum is integrated and comprehensive.

Principle: Holistic Approach Through Integrated, Comprehensive Services Whenever Possible

The holistic approach to assessment and care is best suited to addressing the health behaviors, concerns, and problems of young people, as the risks and vulnerabilities they face are multifaceted and highly interrelated. For example, among U.S. high school students, almost 53 percent engage in two or more risk behaviors, almost 36 percent engage in three or more, and 24 percent engage in four or more (Fox et al., 2010). Most telling, however, is how interrelated risk factors are in terms of poor outcomes. For example, of those (10 percent) whose last intercourse was unprotected, 43.5 percent reported persistent sadness, 41.5 percent reported suicidal thoughts and plans, and 45.9 percent reported problem alcohol behavior. Though, in contrast to studies of adolescents, there are few studies of young adults, many engage in multiple, interrelated risk behaviors (Galambos and Tilton-Weaver, 1998). Clearly, in working with young people, a health provider must assess across a broad range of physical, behavioral, and psychosocial domains. This challenges us to think about young people's physical health, sexual and reproductive health, and emotional well-being in a highly connected and coordinated way (Woods and Neinstein, 2002), and if we identify an area of risk, to ask about other risks and vulnerabilities.

Young people can be extremely sensitive to the perceptions of others, including their peers, and will often forego care if there is risk of shame and embarrassment (Huppert et al., 2003). If comprehensive services are available only through collaborations with other service providers or by collocating services, the way they are coordinated and the referral process should be stigma free. At MSAHC, having all services under one roof and as part of an integrated center makes this much easier to accomplish. Because the way services are named or scheduled can inadvertently contribute to stigma (e.g., the names "HIV services," "sexual assault services," "mental health," and "family planning" reveal the reason for a young person's visit to others), we ask "Can a person's reason for a visit be identified by other patients in the waiting room?" Having services that are integrated in a physical environment communicates diversity and masks the reasons for any given visit, helping avoid stigma associated with certain concerns.

Principle: Confidentiality

The Society for Adolescent Health and Medicine's Position Paper states that confidentiality is a cornerstone of health care for adolescents under the age of 18 (Ford et al., 2004), and they need to be actively reassured about confidentiality before they will talk openly about issues (Ford et al., 1997). It matters to young adults, too, because adolescent and young-adult health involves highly personal and sensitive subjects—such as the developing body, sexuality, sex, trauma, or behavioral risks, as well as insecurities and worries about what is normal. All young people, including young adults, need assurance that they can talk confidentially with their provider (Ford et al., 1997), or they may forego care if they are not reassured about privacy and confidentiality (Ginsberg et al., 1995; Klein et al., 1999). Confidentiality laws level the field so all young people can get the services they need, rather than elect not to get necessary care because they fear disappointing adults in their lives or because they fear recrimination. However, physicians too commonly do not discuss confidentiality with adolescents, and so adolescents are generally unaware of their rights to confidential services (Lehrer et al., 2007; McKee et al., 2001).

Young adults who are covered by a parent or guardian's private insurance plan may also have concerns about the reason for their visit being disclosed by an EOB sent to the policyholder when they have used services for sensitive issues. At MSAHC, patients who do not wish to use a parent's insurance plan are not billed, but for many health providers, an effort to fundraise to cover the costs of services may not be viable. This can be properly addressed only if changes are made to the current practice of sending an EOB to the primary policyholder.

At MSAHC, an adolescent- and young-adult-sensitive consent-to-care process helps ensure confidentiality not just for sexual and reproductive health care but also to secure informational, social, psychological, and physical privacy. Ensuring that the care model is supportive of one-on-one youth–provider interactions is a key element of confidential care, and it encourages young people to freely share their concerns. This requires that staff are competent and comfortable in negotiating this confidential space, for instance, asking parents to wait in the waiting room prior to taking a history and reassuring them that they will be invited back in after the physical examination to discuss any remaining issues after a confidential interview with the young person.

Principle: Provider Preparation, Comfort, and Communication

A final set of considerations for ensuring youth-friendly care relates to provider comfort and competencies. Research suggests that clinician-related barriers to adolescent care include provider insensitivity (Ford et al., 1999); insufficient/inadequate communication (Lim et al., 2012); lack of comfort, knowledge, and skills regarding sexual and reproductive health; discomfort with discussion of sexual behavior with adolescents (IOM, 2009); and lack of time to spend with each patient (McKee et al., 2001). Young people require a relationship-based approach because they place a higher importance on the personal characteristics of their medical provider than adults (Fox et al., 2010). Working with young people is best done by those who like adolescents and have adolescent-specific training, so at MSAHC, care is mostly provided by adolescent specialists, and a great deal of emphasis is placed on interdisciplinary collaboration and cooperation. Having well-trained staff helps in building a culture in which young people are dealt with respectfully, in a nonjudgmental way, and are supported in learning to make their own decisions. Although there are no recent studies as to what type of provider provides adolescents with health care, past studies have shown that most adolescents are seen by general pediatricians or family practitioners (Rand et al., 2007) and, given the low number of adolescent medicine physicians across the country, the field of adolescent health is faced with significant resource limitations.

CONCLUSION

The service-design-and-delivery recommendations presented here will not provide solutions to all health disparities faced by adolescents and young adults. Poor health outcomes related to the relationship between health status and poorer education (Winkleby et al., 1992), criminal-system racial disparities (Iguch et al., 2005), or rural versus urban residence require broader social solutions. Nevertheless, we believe that adolescent- and young-adult-friendly health services, such as

MSAHC, provide tremendous opportunities to better understand how many disparities related to lack of access, poor-quality services, or services that are inadequate because they are not designed to engage young people and sustain them in care might be addressed.

REFERENCES

Advocates for Youth. 2017. *Best practices for youth friendly services: An overview.* Available from http://www.advocatesforyouth.org/publications/publications-a-z/1347--best-practices-for-youth-friendly-clinical-services.

Alexander, S. C., J. D. Fortenberry, K. I. Pollak, T. Bravender, J. K. Davis, T. Ostbye, J. A. Tulsky, R. J. Dolor, and C. G. Shields. 2014. Sexuality talk during adolescent health maintenance visits. *JAMA Pediatrics* 168(2):163–169.

AHRQ (Agency for Healthcare Research and Quality). 2017. *Defining the PCMH.* Available from https://www.pcmh.ahrq.gov/page/defining-pcmh.

American Academy of Pediatrics. 2016. *The medical home.* Available from https://medicalhomeinfo.aap.org/overview/Pages/Whatisthemedicalhome.aspx.

Ames. N. 2008. Medically underserved children's access to health care: A review of the literature. *Journal of Human Behavior in the Social Environment* 18(1):64–77.

Blum, R. W., T. Beuhring, M. Wunderlich, and M. D. Resnick. 1996. Don't ask, they won't tell: The quality of adolescent health screening in five practice settings. *American Journal of Public Health* 86(12):1767–1772.

Blum, W. M., and L. H. Bearlinger. 1990. Knowledge and attitudes of health professionals toward adolescent health care. *Journal of Adolescent Health Care* 11:289–294.

Brown, S. L., J. A. Teufel, and D. A. Birch. 2007. Early adolescents' perceptions of health and health literacy. *Journal of School Health* 77(1):7–15.

Burton, C. M., M. P. Marshall, D. J. Chisolm, G. S. Sucato, and M. S. Friedman. 2013. Sexual minority-related victimization as a mediator of mental health disparities in sexual minority youth: A longitudinal analysis. *Journal of Youth and Adolescence* 42:394–402.

Catalano, R. F., M. L. Bergland, J. M. Ryan, H. S. Lonczak, and J. D. Hawkins. 2004. Positive youth development in the United States: Research findings on evaluations of positive youth development programs. *Annals of the American Academy of Political and Social Science* 591:98–124.

Centers for Medicare & Medicaid Services. 2016. *The Center for Consumer Information & Insurance Oversight.* Available from https://www.cms.gov/CCIIO/Resources/Files/adult_child_fact_sheet.html.

Claxton, G., M. Rae, N. Panchal, A. Damico, H. Whitmore, K. Kenward, and A. Osei-Anto. 2012. Health benefits in 2012: Moderate premium increases for employer-sponsored plans; young adults gained coverage under ACA. *Health Affairs* 31(10).

Diaz, A., K. Peake, M. Surko, and K. Bhandarkar. 2005. Including "at-risk" adolescents in their own health and mental health care: A Youth Development perspective. *Social Work in Mental Health* 3(1–2):3–22.

Eccles, J. S., C. Midgely, A. Wigfield, C. M. Buchanan, D. Reuman, C. Flanagan, and D. MacIver. 1993. Development during adolescence: The impact of stage-environment fit on young adolescents' experiences in schools and in families. *American Psychologist* 48(2):90–101.

Elster, A., J. Jarosik, J. VanGeest, and M. Fleming. 2003. Racial and ethnic disparities in health care for adolescents: A systematic review of the literature. *Archives of Pediatric and Adolescent Medicine* 157:867–874.

Fiscella, K., and D. R. Williams. 2004. Health disparities based on socioeconomic inequities: Implications for urban health care. *Academic Medicine* 79:1139–1147.

Ford, C., A. English, and G. Sigman. 2004. Confidential health care for adolescents: Position paper of the Society for Adolescent Medicine. *Journal of Adolescent Health* 35:160–167.

Ford C. A., P. Bearman, and J. Moody. 1999. Foregone health care among adolescents. *Journal of the American Medical Association* 282(23):2227–2234.

Ford, C., S. Millstein, B. Halpern-Felsher, and C. J. Irwin. 1997. Influence of physician confidentiality assurances on adolescents' willingness to disclose information and seek future health care. A randomized controlled trial. *Journal of the American Medical Association* 278(12):1029–1034.

Fox, H. B., M. A. McManus, C. E. Irwin, Jr., K. J. Kelleher, and K. Peake. 2013. A research agenda for adolescent-centered primary care in the United States. *Journal of Adolescent Health* 53(3):307–310.

Fox, H. B., M. A. McManus, J. D. Klein, A. Diaz, A. B. Elster, M. E. Felice, D. W. Kaplan, C. J. Wibbelsman, and J. E. Wilson. 2010. Adolescent Medicine Training in Pediatric Residency Programs. *Pediatrics* 125(1):165–172.

Fox, H. B., M. A. McManus, and A. G. Michelman. 2013. *Many low income older adolescents likely to remain uninsured in 2014*. National Alliance to Advance Adolescent Health, Fact Sheet 10.

Fox, H. B., S. G. Philliber, M. A. McManus, and S. M. Yurkiewicz. 2010. *Adolescents' experiences and views on health care*. The National Alliance to Advance Adolescent Health, Washington, DC.

Galambos, N. L., and L. C. Tilton-Weaver. 1998. Multiple-risk behavior in adolescents and young adults. *Health Reports* 10. Available from http://www.statcan.gc.ca/pub/82-003-x/1998002/article/3992-eng.pdf.

Ginsberg, K., G. Slap, A. Cnaan, C. C. Forke, C. M. Bellesly, and D. M. Rouselle. 1995. Adolescents' perceptions of factors influencing their decisions to seek health care. *Journal of the American Medical Association* 273:1913–1918.

Gray, N. J., J. D. Klein, P. R. Noyce, T. S. Sesselberg, and J. A. Cantrill. 2005. Health information-seeking behaviour in adolescence: The place of the Internet. *Social Science & Medicine* 60(7):1467–1478.

Gold, R., B. Kennedy, F. Connell, and I. Kawachi. 2002. Teen births, income inequality, and social capital: Developing an understanding of the causal pathway. *Health Place* 8:77–83.

Harper, G. W., D. Lemos, and S. G. Hosek. 2014. Stigma reduction in adolescents and young adults newly diagnosed with HIV: Findings from the Project ACCEPT Intervention. *AIDS Patient Care and STDs* 28(10):543–554.

Health Care Cost Institute. 2014. *Selected health care trends for young adults (ages 19–25)*. Issue Brief #8. Available from http://www.healthcostinstitute.org/files/IB8_YA_09242014.pdf.

Hudson, D. L., E. Puterman, K. Bibbins-Domingo, K. A. Matthews, and N. E. Adler. 2013. Race, life course, socioeconomic position, racial discrimination, depressive symptoms and self-rated health. *Social Science & Medicine* 97:7–14.

Huppert, J. S., and P. K. Adams-Hillard. 2003. Sexually transmitted disease screening in teens. *Current Women's Health Report* 2:451–458.

Iguch, M. Y., J. Bell, R. N. Ramchand, and T. Fain. 2005. How criminal-system racial disparities may translate into health disparities. *Journal of Care for the Poor and Underserved* 16:48–56.

Institute of Medicine (IOM) and National Research Council (NRC). 2009. *Adolescent health services: Missing opportunities.* Washington, DC: The National Academies Press.

IOM and NRC. 2014. *Investing in the health and well-being of young adults.* Washington, DC: The National Academies Press.

Irwin, C. E., S. H. Adams, M. J. Park, and P. W. Newacheck. 2009. Preventive care for adolescents: Few get visits and fewer get services. *Pediatrics* 123:e565e72.

Klein, J., and K. Wilson. 2002. Delivering quality health care: Discussion of adolescents' health risks with their providers. *Journal of Adolescent Health* 30:190–195.

Klein, J., K. Wilson, M. McNulty, C. Kapphahn, and C. S. Collins. 1999. Access to medical care for adolescents: Results from the 1997 Commonwealth Fund Survey of the Health of Adolescent Girls. *Journal of Adolescent Health* 25:120–130.

Larson, R. W. 2000. Toward a psychology of positive youth development. *American Journal of Psychology* 55(1):170–183.

Lehrer, J. A., R. Pantell, K. Tebb, and M. A. Shafer. 2007. Foregone health care among US adolescents: Associations between risk characteristics and confidentiality concern. *Journal of Adolescent Health* 40(3):218–226.

Lim, S. W., R. Chhabra, A. Rosen, A. D. Racine, and E. M. Alderman. 2012. Adolescents' views on barriers to health care: A Pilot Study. *Journal of Primary Care and Community Care* 3(2):99–103.

McKee, M. D., S. E. Rubin, G. Campos, and L. F. O'Sullivan. 2001. Challenges of providing confidential care to adolescents in urban primary care: Clinician perspectives. *Annals of Family Medicine* 9(1):37–43.

McManus, M. A., and H. B. Fox. 2007. *Making the case for addressing adolescent health care.* Washington, DC: National Alliance to Advance Adolescent Health.

McNeely, C., and J. Blanchard. 2009. *The teen years explained: A guide to healthy adolescent development.* Baltimore, MD: Johns Hopkins Bloomberg School of Public Health, Center for Adolescent Health.

Manganello, J. A. 2009. *Health literacy and adolescents: An agenda for the future.* Available from http://www.neahin.org/healthliteracy/Images/Manganello%20Paper.pdf.

Miech, R. A., S. A. Kumanyika, N. Stettler, B. G. Link, J. Phelan, and V. W. Chang. 2006. Trends in the association of poverty with overweight among US adolescents, 1971–2004. *Journal of the American Medical Association* 295 (20):2385–2393.

Mount Sinai Adolescent Health Center. 2016. *Mission statement.* Available from http://www.teenhealthcare.org/all-about-us/who-we-are.

Mount Sinai Adolescent Health Center. 2017. *Blueprint for adolescent and young adult Healthcare.* Available from http://www.teenhealthcare.org/wp-content/uploads/sites/7/2017/01/MSAHC-Blueprint-Guide_v11-Web-2-FINAL.compressed.pdf.

Mulye, T. P., M. J. Park, C. D. Nelson, S. H. Adams, C. E. Irwin, and C. D. Brindis. 2009. Trends in adolescent and young adult health in the United States. *Journal of Adolescent Health* 45(1):8–24.

National Conference of State Legislatures. 2011. *The Affordable Care Act: Implications for adolescents and young adults.* Available from http://www.ncsl.org/portals/1/documents/health/HRAdolescents.pdf.

Neumark-Sztainer, D., M. Story, P. J. Hannan, and J. Croll. 2002. Ethnic/racial differences in weight-related concerns and behaviors among adolescent girls and boys: Findings from Project EAT. *Research and Practice* 29(5):844–851.

Newacheck, P. W., J. M. Park, C. D. Brindis, M. Biehl, and C. E. Irwin. 2004. Trends in Private and Public Health Insurance for Adolescents. *Journal of the American Medical Association* 291(10):1231–1237.

Office of Disease Prevention and Health Promotion. 2016. Available from https://www.healthypeople.gov/2020/topics-objectives/topic/Adolescent-Health?topicid=2#Ref_01.

Peake, K., I. Epstein, and D. Medeiros. 2005. *What kids need to talk about: Clinical and research uses of an adolescent intake questionnaire.* Binghamton, NY: Haworth Press.

Pittman, K., M. Irby, and T. Ferber. 2000. Unfinished business: Further reflections on a decade of promoting youth development. In *Youth development: Issues, challenges and directions.* Philadelphia, PA: Public/Private Ventures.

Rand, C. M., L. P. Shone, C. Albertin, P. Auinger, J. D. Klein, and P. G. Szilagyi. 2007. National health care visit patterns of adolescents: Implications for delivery of new adolescent vaccines. *Archives of Pediatric & Adolescent Medicine* 161:252–259.

Reddy, D. M., R. Fleming, and C. Swain. 2002. Effect of mandatory parental notification on adolescent girls' use of sexual health care services. *Journal of the American Medical Association* 288(7):10–14.

Resnick, M. D., R. W. Blum, and D. Hedin. 1980. The appropriateness of health services for adolescent youths' opinions and attitudes. *Journal of Adolescent Health Care* 1:137–141.

Rural Health Association. 2016. *Rural mental health.* Available from https://www.ruralhealthinfo.org/topics/mental-health.

Saewyc, E. M. 2011. Research on adolescent sexual orientation: Development, health disparities, stigma and resilience. *Journal of Research on Adolescence* 21(1):256–272.

Scales, P. C., and N. Leffert. 1999. *Developmental assets: A synthesis of the scientific research on adolescent development.* Minneapolis, MN: Search Institute.

Schoen, C., K. Davis, K. Scott Collins, L. Greenberg, C. Des Roches, and M. Abrams. 1997. *The Commonwealth Fund survey of the health of adolescent girls.* New York: The Commonwealth Fund.

Schuster, M. A., R. M. Bell, L. P. Petersen, and D. E. Kanouse. 1996. Communication between adolescents and physicians about sexual behavior and risk prevention. *Archives of Pediatric and Adolescent Medicine* 150(9):906–913.

Schuster, M. A., M. N. Elliott, D. E. Kanouse, J. L. Wallander, S. R. Tortolero, J. A. Ratner, D. J. Klein, P. M. Cuccaro, S. L. Davies, and S. W. Banspach. 2012. Racial and ethnic health disparities among fifth-graders in three cities. *New England Journal of Medicine* 367(8):735–745.

Sia, C., T. F. Tonniges, E. Osterhus, and S. Taba. 2004. History of the medical home concept. *Pediatrics* 113(5 Suppl):1473-1478.

Singh, G. K., M. D. Kogan, and P. C. van Dyck. 2008. A multi-level analysis of state and regional disparities in childhood and adolescent obesity in the United States. *Journal of Community Health* 33:90–102.

Stille, C., R. M. Turchi, R. Antonelli, M. D. Cabana, T. L. Cheng, D. Laraque, and J. Perrin. 2010. The family-centered medical home: Specific considerations for child health research and policy. *Academic Pediatrics.* Available from http://www.nihcm. org/pdf/Attachment_B_-APA_Article_FCMH.pdf.

Surko, M., D. Ciro, E. Carlson, N. Labor, V. Giannone, E. Diaz-Cruz, K. Peake, and I Epstein. 2005. Which adolescents need to talk about safety and violence? *Social Work in Mental Health* 3(1–2):103–120.

U.S. Census Bureau. 2016. *Annual estimates of the resident population for selected age groups by sex for the United States, states, counties, and Puerto Rico Commonwealth and municipios: April 1, 2010 to July 1, 2015.* Available from https://factfinder.census.gov/faces/tableservices/jsf/pages/productview.xhtml?src=bkmk.

U.S. Department of Agriculture (USDA). 2015. *Rural America at a glance.* Available from http://www.ers.usda.gov/media/1952235/eib145.pdf.

U.S. Department of Health and Human Services (HHS). *The changing face of America's adolescents.* Available from http://www.hhs.gov/ash/oah/adolescenthealth-topics/americas-adolescents/changing-face.html.

Vo, D. X., and M. J. Park. 2008. Racial/ethnic disparities and culturally competent health care among youth and young men. *American Journal of Men's Health* 2:192–205.

Walker, I., M. McManus, and H. Fox. 2011. *Medical home innovations: Where do adolescents fit?* Washington, DC: National Alliance to Advance Adolescent Health.

Winkleby, M. A., D. E. Jatulis, E. Frank, and S. P. Fortmann. 1992. Socioeconomic status and health: how education, income, and occupation contribute to risk factors for cardiovascular disease. *American Journal of Public Health* 82(6):816–820.

Woods, E., and L. Neinstein. 2002. Office visit techniques and recommendations to parents. In *Adolescent health care: A practical guide.* New York: Lippincott, Williams and Wilkins.

Youngblade, L. M., C. Theokas, J. Schulenber, L. Curry, I. Huang, and M. Novak. 2007. Risk and promotive factors in families, schools, and communities: A contextual model of positive youth development. *Adolescence* 119 (Suppl 1):S47–S53.

ACKNOWLEDGMENTS

The authors would like to acknowledge the Evaluation Team at ICF International for their effort in studying and iterating the principles of adolescent- and young-adult-friendly care and operation embedded in the design and delivery of services at the Mount Sinai Adolescent Health Center. They are Christine Walrath, Gingi Pica, Lisa Carver, and Cathy Lesesne.

SECTION III: ADVANCING HEALTH EQUITY IN COMMUNITIES OF COLOR

9

STORIES ABOUT BLACK MEN IN THE MEDIA AND THEIR CONSEQUENCES FOR HEALTH

Karen E. Dill-Shackleford, PhD, Srividya Ramasubramanian, PhD, MA, and Lawrence M. Drake II, PhD, MA, MPA

At this particular juncture in U.S. history, the fictional entertainment and news media stories we tell about black men are vitally important to our individual and collective development as a society. Mainstream media frequently reproduce white racial frames by presenting white characters as normal and superior to characters of color in narratives and entertainment. In the media, black men are overrepresented as street criminals (Burgess et al., 2011; Dill and Burgess, 2012; Dixon and Linz, 2000; Lacy and Haspel, 2011) and under-represented in positive social roles (Burgess et al., 2011) and in positions of power (Turner, 2014). Even when present within media narratives, black men are often relegated to the background (Wilkes and Valencia, 1989). A number of studies have demonstrated that the stories we tell about black men in the media have negative consequences such as increased prejudice and decreased support for pro-black ideas and policies (Behm-Morawitz and Ortiz, 2013; Dill and Burgess, 2012; Mastro, 2003; Ramasubramanian, 2010). On the positive side, progressive portrayals or counterstereotypes have been shown to result in more positive outcomes and attitudes related to black men (Dill and Burgess, 2012; Ramasubramanian, 2007, 2011; Scharrer and Ramasubramanian, 2015). We discuss these studies and others, in this chapter, and put them in context of current events in the United States related to the role of black men in society. One facet of current racial and ethnic tensions that is crucial to understand is that racism in its many forms, including that perpetuated in media, is related to negative psychological and physical health outcomes.

The most prominent of contemporary stories about black males in the media relate to the Black Lives Matter (BLM) movement. The BLM movement arose after a series of events involving mistreatment or mishandling of, or violence toward, African Americans by white police officers and other authorities. The movement began after George Zimmerman, a white adult, was acquitted after shooting Trayvon Martin, an African American teenager, and also in response to the killing of unarmed African American teenager Michael Brown in Ferguson, Missouri, by white police officer Darren Wilson. During a vigil with the Browns and civil rights activist Rev. Al Sharpton in New York City, the Brown family lawyer questioned what he called a public habit of vilifying black children while putting whites on a pedestal.

It was BLM, aided by a savvy social media campaign identifying itself via the Twitter hashtag #BlackLivesMatter, that broke through the media clutter to establish a coherent voice and a mobilization effort that rallied communities across the country about the social and racial significance of Trayvon Martin's death. BLM's activist efforts were further fueled by outrage among many black Americans after the subsequent shootings of black men by white men such as Michael Brown in Ferguson, Missouri, and later of Philando Castille near St. Paul, Minnesota. These recent shootings involving mostly white law enforcement officers summoned recollections of the deaths of other black men whose lives ended during the black struggle for civil rights in the 1960s, such as Jimmie Lee Jackson, shot just after a planning meeting on voter registration in Selma, Alabama, or Samuel Hammond Jr., Henry Smith, and Delano Middleton, students at South Carolina State University who were shot and killed during a peaceful protest against a local, segregated bowling alley. The BLM movement also offered a perspective on how to plot the use of technology-based communication platforms to expose the injustice of the violence being perpetrated while unifying their message.

These stories and their dissemination via mass media highlight burning social issues about the place in society of African American boys and men, and their families and communities. They speak to children and parents everywhere about a larger understanding of the intersection of social identities such as race and gender and how they influence the individual's status in society.

STORIES ABOUT BLACK MEN IN THE MEDIA

Historically, media have presented black males in a stereotypical and unfavorable light as violence prone, criminal, lazy, unintelligent, and buffoonish (Berkowitz, 2008; Bogle, 2001; Dixon and Linz, 2000; Stroman et al., 1989). It is outside the scope of this article to review a complete history of stereotypes of African Americans in the media. However, one historical example may help put this in context: Entman and Rojecki (2001) reference a historical advertisement published in March 1796 in a newspaper in Charleston, South Carolina: the *City Gazette*. The advertisement read, "Fifty Prime Negroes for sale on Tuesday the 15th of March." The ad completed its description by indicating "the wenches are young and improving; the boys, girls and children are remarkably smart. Fitted for either house or plantation work" (Mehlinger, 1970, p. 129). While the descendants of those mentioned in this advertisement are no longer referred to as Negroes and instead are recognized interchangeably as blacks or African Americans, their media portrayals continue to be steeped in symbolic racism, arguably not too different from the image projected in this ad published 200 years ago (Entman and Rojecki, 2001).

MEDIA STEREOTYPES OF BLACK MEN

Although there has been an increase in portrayals of African American men in media stories in present-day contexts, the representations continue to be negative and stereotypical. Within news–reporting contexts, for instance, scholars continue to document ways racial coding impacts racial attitudes and behaviors (Dixon, 2015; Dixon and Linz, 2000; Entman and Rojecki, 2001). News reports often use subtle cues and visual codes that rationalize white superiority and present black men as disruptive and troublesome. Beyond portraying black males in stereotypical ways, news stories also play a role in implicitly influencing audiences' perceptions of why racial inequalities exist in society. Research documents that news stories about black men often attribute their failures to personal deficiencies such as incompetence or lack of motivation rather than to systemic factors such as discrimination or lack of access (Pan and Kosicki, 1993; Ramasubramanian, 2010).

In addition to stories in the news media, negative stories about black men from fictional media such as television, film, and video games continue to distort realities about black men and to exert negative influences (Bogle, 2001; Ford, 1997). In video games, for example, there is a tendency to portray men as aggressive in general; however, even there, the story about white men and black men differs (Burgess et al., 2011). Whereas white men's aggression is presented more often as socially sanctioned (e.g., police and soldiers), black men's aggression is presented as being criminal and dangerous. The reality of black men as policemen and soldiers is a story that's not told here. The story that is told is one of black men as the dangerous minority, brandishing extreme weapons (Burgess et al., 2011).

While white males were overrepresented and black males were underrepresented in this study on video games, black men were more likely to be shown as fighting than white men and white men were far more likely to be depicted using technology (implying perhaps intelligence and/or affluence) than black men. Not a single black man was represented as a soldier in this sample, which is not in sync with reality. Interestingly, white men were much more likely than black men to be shown wearing protective armor. Taken together, this is indeed a negative and judgmental story about black men, suggesting that black men are violent, commit crimes, have disproportionately powerful bodies, and do not need armor to protect themselves when compared with whites. It has also been shown that, in video games, mere exposure to black male characters evokes greater aggressive thoughts than does exposure to white male characters among white players (Burgess et al., 2011). The authors interpreted these differences as likely being caused by the idea that black men are seen as threatening and aggressive. The black male body had become symbolic of violence (Dill and Burgess, 2012).

COUNTERSTEREOTYPES AND POSITIVE MEDIA PORTRAYALS

Recent research suggests that while stereotypes in the media can negatively influence audiences, representations that run counter to stereotypes, or "counterstereotypes" (also referred to as "countertypes"), can reduce prejudice (see, e.g., Holt, 2013; Ramasubramanian, 2011, 2015). For example, representations of black men as kind and law abiding in contrast to typical stereotypes of being violence prone and criminal would be counterstereotypes. Research on positive exemplars (prototypical examples of a case) and on countertypes (counterstereotypical images and stories) both indicate the need for change in our portrayal of black men and the positive consequences promised by such change. For example, likely because of the attributions made when one violates expectations positively, positive exemplars of black men have been rated more highly than positive exemplars of white men (Dill and Burgess, 2012). On the other end of the spectrum, negative exemplars of black men are rated less favorably than negative exemplars of black men (Dill and Burgess, 2012).

When white audiences' form emotional bonds through fictional narratives and media stories with admirable black celebrities such as Oprah Winfrey, it can lead to favorable attitudes toward blacks in general, an effect known as *parasocial contact* (Ramasubramanian, 2011, 2015). In another study (Dill and Burgess, 2012), researchers investigated the difference that exposure to stereotypical versus counterstereotypical portrayals of African American men made on pro-black attitudes and on reactions toward either a white or a black male political candidate with the same credentials. After viewing stereotypical images, a black male candidate was rated less favorably than a white male candidate with the same credentials. In contrast, after viewing counterstereotypical images, the black male candidate was rated more favorably than the white male candidate. These differences held for ratings of global favorability, capability, and likability, and even for behavioral intentions to vote for a particular candidate.

The premise of such research, based on the priming paradigm, is that simply bringing to mind a stereotype or a counterstereotype is sufficient to influence subsequent judgments, beliefs, and behavioral intentions. Taken together, these research results indicate that exposure to stereotypes influences beliefs and intentions toward black men negatively while exposure to counterstereotypes influences these same outcomes positively. In the long run, one very important question is the relative availability of stereotypical cultural representations of black men as compared to the availability of counterstereotypes. The hope is that adequate counterstereotypical representation will improve social outcomes and also reduce the effects of dominant cultural stereotypes themselves. This body of scholarship makes a case for the need for diverse and complex portrayals of black men in the media.

MEANING MAKING AND AUDIENCE RESPONSES

Ours is not a hypodermic model of media exposure. In other words, human beings do not react like automatons to the content they view, but bring with them experiences, emotions, and beliefs that shape their perceptions, understanding, and responses to mediated stories. In fact, fictional narratives evoke strong emotions and can be a forum for working out personal social issues (see, e.g., Oatley, 1999). Thus, the experience differs from person to person. We ask: What difference do the stories about black men from our shared culture make to black men and to others?

Because media are often seen as trivial, our exposure to the stories media tell—for example, stories about black men—are also seen as trivial. This is perhaps due, in part, to a common belief that entertainment media are primarily sources of simple, hedonic enjoyment. In simple terms, media viewing is just for fun and therefore not meaningful. However, the latest research in media psychology calls this perspective into question (e.g., Oliver and Bartsch, 2011). While some media experiences are undoubtedly light and fun, others have much more depth and consequence. In the case of the stories we tell about black men, as we have seen here, the stories we entertain in the culture influence not only how black males see themselves, but how others see black males.

In terms of how such stories impact blacks themselves, studies such as those conducted by Parker and Moore (2014) provide important insights. These scholars conducted a qualitative study on African American college males' perceptions of their own representation in the media. Their findings uncovered two relevant themes. One is that the respondents were highly aware of the prevalence of the negative portrayals, particularly of black males, in both digital and traditional media. The second major theme was the idea that America has evolved to a postracial society (an era without racism or discrimination) is a fallacy (Parker and Moore, 2014).

Exposure to negative stereotypes in the media, especially by heavier consumers of media, leads to the formation of entrenched stereotypes by white audiences about black men, which extend from beliefs to policy opinions of viewers (Abraham and Appiah, 2006; Armstrong et al., 1992; Dixon and Azocar, 2007; Tan et al., 2000). Even subtle cues in media that stereotype black men can be sufficient to activate both explicit and implicit biases. Explicit bias refers to conscious endorsement of stereotypes whereas implicit bias refers to subtle judgments that operate at the subconscious level. Such media cues lead to misidentification of criminal suspects as black, and lead to lesser support for pro-minority policies such as affirmative action (Oliver and Fonash, 2002; Ramasubramanian, 2011). These effects are especially strong when direct face-to-face contact is absent between racial groups (Fujioka, 1999; Ramasubramanian, 2013). These negative stories of black males in the media also have detrimental self-stereotyping effects on blacks themselves (Fujioka, 2005). Exposure to these negative portrayals can reduce black men's self-esteem and self-efficacy (Opportunity Agenda, 2012). Furthermore, we know that there are racial differences in criminal sentencing that result in disproportional numbers of black men getting the death penalty. Also, police simulations indicate that black men are disproportionately more likely than white men to be shot in these scenarios (Opportunity Agenda, 2012).

Box 9-1 tells the story of how the image of black men affected the experience of one young black man, Martese Johnson. Johnson experienced firsthand violent treatment and the frustration of others mistaking who they think you are because you are a black man (more on that and on possible solutions in Box 9-1). Now, we turn to the particular topic of black men's health and tie it to cultural stereotypes that are often propagated by the media.

MEDIA AND AFRICAN AMERICAN HEALTH OUTCOMES

The stigmatization of black men extends to the health domain because media disseminate stories and ideas about black men that have consequences, as described above. Prejudice and discrimination, which are psychological factors and, in part,

BOX 9-1
On the Need to Amplify Black Male Voices

In spring 2014 on a cool March evening, a news video of a young man being savagely beaten and berated by white officers of the Virginia Alcoholic Beverage and Control Unit near the campus of the University of Virginia gave rise to the anger of frustration of yet another negative portrayal of a black male that so often begins the news cycles of American media. While the disgusting sight of this young black man lying in the street bleeding and pleading with these officers to stop striking him, while shouting "I didn't do anything," was almost unwatchable, the third author of this essay had to continue to fight the anguished thought that this is who the police think all black men are: criminals.

The voice of this story is that of a black man who has experienced a range of social identities: from homeless boy to a Fortune 500 senior executive featured on the cover of the *Wall Street Journal* to a research scholar. The precarious challenge that the third author often faces when describing the potpourri of his experiences ranging from aspiration and joy to outright disrespect, is which story does he tell and how can he describe his experiences in a manner that speaks to the internal confidence he has to have to survive, while also sharing the pain and anxiety of constantly being confronted with images and narratives of negativity that encourage inferiority.

The author of this story is keenly aware that whites generally view his improbable journey through the subtle but powerful lens of "exceptionalism." In other words, his outcomes are supposedly different from those of other black males. However, on this night, viewing the brutality forced upon the young man, Martese, was akin to watching himself live. The connection he felt as he watched each blow being landed by these officers was as if he was being struck too.

As the President/CEO of the LEADership, Education, and Development program (often referred to as LEAD), the nation's foremost youth talent development and education advocacy organization, the author's connection to Martese Johnson went beyond being of the same race and gender. Martese was a 2008 graduate of LEAD's engineering program that is conducted in partnership with the University of Virginia.

The goal of LEAD is to encourage diverse young men and women of color to prepare and apply for, and graduate from, the most well-known colleges and universities around the world. Since its inception over 35 years ago, over

10,000 young people of color have matriculated through this program. The college graduation rate for those out of this program is also an impressive 99.7 percent. Additionally, approximately 41 percent of those who attend the summer institutes and year-round engagement activities in business, engineering, and computer science are black and fully 45–50 percent are male.

Black males such as Martese Johnson and the author are deeply committed to access for blacks to education, which they see as a vital factor in influencing psychosocial progress of black males in American society. Despite LEAD's transformative learning agenda, its world-class, experiential, summer residency program, and life preparation activities, preparing black youth for the media stereotypes that often define them in larger social contexts remains a big challenge.

Despite the progress of black males in education, industry, and other areas of America's landscape, media continue to highlight a negative narrative that associates black men with violence, crime, and poverty. In other words, the image of a black president and the bloody face of Martese Johnson are not opposite, but represent two visuals that are perceived in the same manner by the white majority. It is time for the media to report the true story—not the outdated stereotypes we view all day every day.

born of cultural transmissions, are factors in racial health disparities (Stuber et al., 2008). In the *Lancet*, Wailoo (2006) details how, historically, media have sent cultural messages about African Americans as disease carriers and as toxic to whites. Cultural messages can foster prejudice, which results in health disparities for the stigmatized group.

It remains vitally important to note that, over time, racial differentiation has been heavily influenced by what has been noticed, processed, interpreted, and remembered and even discarded about blacks in America. The racial status quo exists with whites at the apex of most American institutions and racial minorities at or near the bottom, overrepresented among the poor, and underrepresented in positions within government, higher education, corporate leadership, and health care (Larson, 2006). The infant mortality rate among blacks is twice that of whites. Black men are seven times more likely than whites to be diagnosed with HIV and more than twice as likely to die of prostate cancer (CDC, 2013).

In 1999, Congress requested a study from the Institute of Medicine on disparities in health care based on racial prejudice. The resulting report was entitled

Unequal Treatment: Confronting Racial and Ethnic Disparities in Health Care (IOM, 2003). The major finding of the report was that racial and ethnic minorities were less likely to get proper medical treatment than nonminorities and that they also received lower-quality health care. Furthermore, a recent study by Anderson and colleagues (2014) concluded that racial discrimination is a major source of stress for black people, and therefore the discrimination experienced by black parents may directly or indirectly affect their parenting skills and ultimately their child's well-being.

A growing number of researchers have argued that pervasive racism, including that fostered by the media, has an adverse impact on the health conditions of blacks and other racial minorities (Williams and Williams-Morris, 2000). Nairn and colleagues (2006) agree that media contribute to marginalizing minorities such as by characterizing groups of people as dangerous and problematic. They argue that, "International literature has established that racism contributes to ill-health of migrants, ethnic minorities, and indigenous peoples. Racism generally negates well-being, adversely affecting physical and psychological health" (Nairn et al., 2006, p. 183). These negative outcomes include mental health deficits (Nairn et al., 2006). Their conclusion is that we should treat racism, including institutional racism fostered by media, as a public health concern. Noting that Canada advocated a movement to change anti-Muslim coverage and that New Zealand called for something similar regarding media coverage of their native Maori people, Nairn and colleagues (2006) called for "media racism" to become its own field of study.

Hodgetts (2006, p. 171) positions media as a source of "shared experience"—in other words, culture. While he, like us, does not construe media effects through a hypodermic model, he postulates that viewers grapple with information they see in the media, including healthy and unhealthy messages, and decide what to do with that information. Hodgetts (2006) discusses the idea that crime and violence reporting and coverage should be considered part of health news, for some of the reasons we have mentioned above. For instance, when we stereotype black men as violent, we not only instill fear in others, but we also evoke stress and resulting negative health outcomes in black men. In other words, when we tell false stories about an entire demographic, we cause stress and ill health and even aggression in not only that demographic, but in others who encounter them. Bottom line: Telling these stories about black men is unhealthy for black men and unhealthy for others in society, both psychologically and physically. Hodgetts and Stolte (2009) cautioned that with regard to race, media deliver both healthy and unhealthy information. This latter conclusion suggests, as we outline here, that media literacy interventions are an important step in healing the physical, mental, and social problems stemming from racism in the media.

On a related note, although media are a part of the problem, they can also be part of the solution. For instance, technology-based, mediated communication is providing improvements in accessing health care information. A 1999 longitudinal study sponsored by the Kaiser Family Foundation investigated the role of media as a health information source (Brodie et al., 1999). The study, which included white, African American, and Latino participants, found that a large majority of the 3,400 interviewed rely heavily on the media compared with other sources for information about health care, with television being the most preferred among African Americans (>50 percent). African American and white respondents were asked to rate their perceptions of the general market and racial representation, and fairness of minority portrayals in the context of health topics being discussed in the media. Blacks specifically reported dissatisfaction with the manner in which media address health problems that affect them and equal levels of dissatisfaction with the way media represent and portray black people and black families in health care–related information.

USING DIGITAL MEDIA TECHNOLOGIES FOR SOCIAL GOOD

Overall, 86 percent of all blacks use the Internet, with 73 percent of them using it as a gateway to engage with social media sites. That number grows to 96 percent when measuring 18- to 24-year-olds according to a Pew Research Center study (Smith, 2013). This report provides two important insights: (1) widespread Internet use by blacks provides access to health care information that may have been unavailable to them in the past through traditional media sources, and (2) younger generations of blacks are more likely to use social media sites for purposes that extend beyond health care.

In addition to having the same historical broadcast channels that have moved from analog to digital formats, media proliferation is in full swing with the growth of cable television, satellite radio, and DirecTV, which offers its subscribers over 700 channels of content including in-demand Hollywood movies (Team, 2015). There are also blogs, social media outlets such as Facebook and Twitter, as well as user-generated content sites such as YouTube and Instagram that all can be accessed using a mobile platform.

With the International Telecommunications Union reporting mobile penetration of 87 percent and a research study conducted by the Pew Research Center

(Smith, 2013) indicating that 92 percent of all African Americans own a mobile phone, mobile computing can become a medium of change for reducing racism and improving the health of black Americans. With greater than 56 percent of mobile phones owned by blacks being smartphone devices, and 19 percent of smartphone owners having at least one health-related app on their smartphone, blacks can have virtually unlimited access to fitness information, specifically, blood pressure, physical activity, and stress, effectively equipping them to address health-related problems, especially those that are often attributed to black culture, without interference or false representation (Smith, 2013).

ALTERNATIVE STORYTELLING FOR BLACK VOICES

Apart from encouraging diverse and positive portrayals of black men in mainstream media, it is important to foster alternative media spaces for black voices to be amplified and heard. One such community-based initiative that directly addresses black masculinity is *Question Bridge* (see Belcher, 2014, and Ramasubramanian, 2015, for more details). This participatory, transmedia, public art project challenges existing stereotypes of black men by providing counternarratives rarely seen in mainstream media. By using over 1,500 microdocumentaries with black men to create a virtual dialogic exchange, Question Bridge provides a rich alternative platform to showcase the complex and fluid identity of black men. Questions range from the everyday mundane to the transcendental and spiritual. This initiative combines the website with other media formats such as geolocation hotspots, mobile applications, live public discussions, museum displays, and virtual street installations to engage audiences in an innovative and interesting way.

When it comes to promoting interracial harmony, another promising method we can harness for improvement is to use new media, including immersive media such as video games and virtual reality, to change hearts and minds. Bachen and colleagues (2012) used a simulation game to enhance intercultural empathy. This game, called *REAL LIVES*, allows players to choose an identity at the intersection of race and gender—for instance, choosing to be a black boy. Their research indicated that pretending to be a character of another race and witnessing that character's experiences and the reactions he received was enough to enhance empathy as well as an interest in learning more about other cultures.

Others have extended this work to virtual reality realms. For example, Groom and colleagues (2009) found that those who had controlled a black avatar in an immersive virtual environment were less apt to show implicit racial bias outside of that environment than those who had controlled a white avatar. These researchers suggest that virtual racial embodiment be used to heighten racial empathy and decrease negative racial attitudes. In a similar study, Peck and colleagues (2013) found that experiencing compelling embodiment of a dark-skinned avatar by light-skinned participants reduced implicit racial bias as measured by the Implicit Association Test.

MEDIA LITERACY AND ANTIRACISM

As concerned citizens and educators, it is important to learn and teach about the ways media stories shape our ideas about the world and ourselves through media literacy education. Anyone with a smartphone or Internet access in the new digital media context is potentially a media "prosumer" who is simultaneously both a *producer* and a *consumer* of media messages. Therefore, media literacy is a crucial lifelong skill to be practiced so we can use media in just, responsible, and inclusive ways. Research shows that media literacy training can reduce racial prejudice and make media users more critical of the ways mainstream media depict racial minorities (Ramasubramanian, 2007; Scharrer and Ramasubramanian, 2015). However, very few media literacy initiatives currently address racial/ethnic stereotypes in their programs.

The role of media in America, and its description and reporting of group action and protest often characterized as *movements,* has both a complicated past and an even more complex present. Numerous examples exist that demonstrate how various media practices over the years attempt to influence audience opinions about the significance of certain social movements from the antiwar campaign to gender equality protest staged by gay and lesbian organizations to the more recent Black Lives Matter movement (Gamson and Modigliani, 1989; Terkildsen and Schnell, 1977).

Gamson and Wolfsfeld (1993) provide additional context and insight into this phenomenon by positing that while media and the nature of movements are somewhat dependent upon one another, the media enjoy the more powerful position. In fact all movements, social or otherwise, must rely on media in three important ways: (1) mobilization of political support, (2) legitimization in the mainstream discourse, and (3) to broaden the conflict. Although Gamson and Wolfsfeld's ideological construct remains important to the success of most movements, the 21st century may ignite a shift in mainstream media's balance of power, due in part to how new mediums and modalities can be used to aid social movements such as the BLM movement in both media creation and message distribution (Barker, 2008).

RESEARCH AGENDA

Given this review of the state of media racism in the United States and its costs to society, both social and health related, we suggest the following research agenda. As outlined above, because media messages are complex, the solution must include a more educated public. A review of the current problems in the U.S. educational system is beyond the scope of this article. Having said that, it is imperative that we find space in our schools to educate our children in media literacy. Such education is not optional; it is critical to being a healthy and productive citizen in our current media-rich climate. Canada knows this and is far ahead of us in media literacy training (e.g., Media Smart Canada [mediasmart.ca]).

Scharrer and Ramasubramanian (2015) reviewed literature on both quantitative and qualitative studies of media literacy interventions for media racism and found that both types of research are rare, but show promise for each type of intervention. We therefore propose that it will be important, moving forward, to follow up on both quantitative and qualitative investigations of the effects of media literacy interventions on race. One important finding that should be considered in future research is the idea that both factors of the message and factors of the audience should be considered when educating people on media literacy (Ramasubramanian, 2007; Scharrer and Ramasubramanian, 2015). The literature on the effectiveness of such interventions is small, so there is much to learn from new tests of interventions. For instance, what aspects of the message and of audience factors are most helpful in reducing prejudice? What instructional aspects (e.g., peer teachers, active learning, and media-based interventions) of the media literacy training make a difference? What is the role of social media in combating media racism?

Qualitative research on media literacy has tended to focus on ethnic minorities as recipients of the interventions (Scharrer and Ramasubramanian, 2015). Results have indicated that minorities can respond to negative stereotypes about themselves with plans to change their own behaviors, sometimes not questioning white privilege (Scharrer and Ramasubramanian, 2015, p. 177). It is important for future work to target the privileged majority and also to target mixed-race groups of students. This would allow for dialogue about responsibility for messaging and for responding to messaging that is derogatory to any one race. Mixed-race groups could be tasked with working together to address the problem. Furthermore, an exploration of the stereotypes present in the school environment and what students, parents, and teachers can do to combat that will be important.

We also suggest more qualitative interviewing with both majority and minority members to learn more about our individual lived experiences with stories about race. The premise, for example, of narrative inquiry (Josselson, 2013) is that the interviewer forms a relationship with the interviewee and then does her best to get out of the way of the interviewee to learn about her lived experience. Another important assumption of this type of narrative inquiry is that the researcher does not know what the participant will say and must be open to hearing what the participant is saying and be resistant to answering the questions posed as she herself would answer.

Thus far we know more about the nature of the messages in the media, mostly via content analysis, than we know about the lived experiences of those who consume the messages. Though we mentioned that most of the narrative inquiries have used minority participants, it is true that most research studies on media effects generally focus on majority participants and the segments of our population who enjoy more privilege. Therefore, we do call for more research that gives voice to minority participants. Since this paper is about black men in particular, we call for more research that gives voice to the lived experience of black men. Questions asked might focus on the stories about their own group that they have perceived as coming from the media. It also may include any experiences where everyday people cite media stories as justification for racism.

Finally, given that we know a skewed representation of black men in the media exists, and given the evidence that negative stereotypes harm and positive images help black men and our society in general, we call for less stereotypical representations of black men in storytelling. A recent example of counterstereotypes in the media would be the main characters in the latest Star Wars film. Finn (a black man) and Rey (a white woman) are friends, are extremely likeable, and are the primary characters of a major motion picture. While some may trivialize the importance of this kind of storytelling, its importance cannot be underestimated.

CONCLUSIONS

Right now, history has made abundantly clear the fact that shared cultural stereotypes of black men are contributing to brutality and injustice toward black men. The subject of police shootings and disproportional imprisonment of black men are frequently in the news. News and entertainment narratives about black men lead to discrimination, to stress, and to negative psychological and physical health consequences that are also taking a disproportionate toll on black men in America. One hundred and fifty years after the Civil War, our inability to offer real equality to black men in the United States is clearly apparent. But, at the same time, with our first African American male completing a second historic term as president, we see that there is cause for optimism. As challenging and distressing as the current state of race relations in the United States is today, social science research points to media as an avenue of hope and change. These avenues include the shared culture of storytelling, news, entertainment, art, and literature. They also extend to new technologies such as a variety of forms of immersive media including virtual reality and video games. Popular media have been part of the problem in racial understanding for years. As we look for opportunities for positive change, there is evidence to suggest that including popular media in the solution is a viable option.

REFERENCES

Abraham, L., and O. Appiah. 2006. Framing news stories: The role of visual imagery in priming racial stereotypes. *Howard Journal of Communications* 17(3):183–203.

Anderson, R. E., S. B. Hussain, M. N. Wilson, D. S. Shaw, T. J. Dishion, and J. L. Williams. 2014. Pathways to pain: Racial discrimination and relations between parental functioning and child psychosocial well-being. *Journal of Black Psychology* 41(6):491–512.

Armstrong, G. B., K. A. Neuendorf, and J. E. Brentar. 1992. TV entertainment, news, and racial perceptions of college students. *Journal of Communication* 42:153–176.

Bachen, C. M., P. F. Hernandez-Ramos, and C. Raphael. 2012. Simulating REAL LIVES: Promoting global empathy and interest in learning through simulation games. *Simulation & Gaming* 43(4):437–460.

Barker, M. 2008. *Mass media and social movements: A critical examination of the relationship between mainstream media and social movements.* Available from www.globalresearch.ca/mass-media-and-social movements/8761.

Behm-Morawitz, E., and M. Ortiz. 2013. *Race, ethnicity, and the media.* Oxford Handbooks Online, doi:10.1093/oxfordhb/9780195398809.013.0014.

Belcher, C. 2014. Question Bridge provides a forum for black men to hold honest discussion. *Style Weekly,* http://www.styleweekly.com/richmond/blackon-black/Content?oid=2097305.

Berkowitz, L. 2008. On the consideration of automatic as well as controlled psychological processes in aggression. *Aggressive Behavior* 34(2):117–129.

Bogle, D. 2001. *Toms, coons, mulattoes, mammies, and bucks: An interpretive history of Blacks in American films.* New York: Continuum.

Brodie, M., N. Kjellson, T. Hoff, and M. Parker. 1999. Perceptions of Latinos, African Americans, and whites on media as a health information source. *Howard Journal of Communications* 10(3):147–167.

Burgess, M. C., K. E. Dill, S. P. Stermer, S. R. Burgess, and B. P. Brown. 2011. Playing with prejudice: The prevalence and consequences of racial stereotypes in video games. *Media Psychology* 14(3):289–311.

CDC (Centers for Disease Control and Prevention). 2013. *National Health Interview Survey.* Available from https://www.cdc.gov/nchs/nhis.

Dill, K. E., and M. C. Burgess. 2012. Influence of black masculinity game exemplars on social judgments. *Simulation & Gaming* 44(4):562–585.

Dixon, T. L. 2015. Good guys are still always in white? Positive change and continued misrepresentation of race and crime on local television news. *Communication Research* 0093650215579223.

Dixon, T. L., and C. L. Azocar. 2007. Priming crime and activating blackness: Understanding the psychological impact of the overrepresentation of blacks as law-breakers on television news. *Journal of Communication* 57(2):229–253

Dixon, T. L., and D. Linz. 2000. Overrepresentation and underrepresentation of African Americans and Latinos as lawbreakers on television news. *Journal of Communication* 50(2):131–154.

Entman, R., and A. Rojecki. 2001. *The black image in the white mind: Media and race in America.* Chicago, IL: University of Chicago Press.

Ford, T. E. 1997. Effects of stereotypical television portrayals of African-Americans on person perception. *Social Psychology Quarterly* 60:266–275.

Fujioka, Y. 1999. Television portrayals and African-American stereotypes: Examination of television effects when direct contact is lacking. *Journalism & Mass Communication Quarterly* 76:52–75.

Fujioka, Y. 2005. Black media images as a perceived threat to African American ethnic identity: Coping responses, perceived public perception, and attitudes towards affirmative action. *Journal of Broadcasting & Electronic Media* 49(4):450–467.

Gamson, W. A., and A. Modigliani. 1989. Media discourse and public opinion on nuclear power: A constructionist approach. *American Journal of Sociology* 95(1):1–37.

Gamson, W. A., and G. Wolfsfeld. 1993. Movements and media as interacting systems. *Annals of the American Academy of Political and Social Science* 528:114–125.

Groom, V., J. N. Bailenson, and C. Nass. 2009. The influence of racial embodiment on racial bias in immersive virtual environments. *Social Influence* 4(3):231–248.

Hodgetts, D. 2006. Media and health: A continuing concern for health psychology. *Journal of Health Psychology* 11(2):171–174.

Hodgetts, D., and O. Stolte. 2009. Questioning "black humour": Facial exploitation, media and health. *Journal of Health Psychology* 14(5):643–646.

Holt, L. F. 2013. Writing the wrong: Can counter-stereotypes offset negative media messages about African Americans? *Journalism & Mass Communication Quarterly* 90(1):108–125.

IOM (Institute of Medicine). 2003. *Unequal treatment: Confronting racial and ethnic disparities in health care.* Washington, DC: The National Academies Press.

Josselson, R. 2013. *Interviewing for qualitative inquiry: A relational approach.* New York: Guilford.

Lacy, M. G., and K. C. Haspel. 2011. Apocalypse: The media's framing of black looters, shooters, and brutes in hurricane Katrina's aftermath. In *Critical rhetorics of race*, edited by M. G. Lacy and K. A. Ono. New York: NYU Press. Pp. 21–46.

Larson S. G. 2006. *Media & minorities: The politics of race in news and entertainment media.* Lanham, MD: Rowman & Littlefield.

Mastro, D. E. 2003. A social identity approach to understanding the impact of television messages. *Communication Monographs* 70(2):98–113.

Mehlinger, K. T. 1970. The image of the black man and the media. *Journal of the National Medical Association.*

Nairn, R., F. Pega, T. McCreanor, J. Rankine, and A. Barnes. 2006. Media, racism and public health psychology. *Journal of Health Psychology* 11(2):183–196.

Oatley, K. 1999. Why fiction may be twice as true as fact: Fiction as cognitive and emotional simulation. *Review of General Psychology* 3(2):101–117.

Oliver, M. B., and A. Bartsch. 2011. Appreciation of entertainment. *Journal of Media Psychology: Theories, Methods, and Applications* 23(1):29–33.

Oliver, M. B., and D. Fonash. 2002. Race and crime in the news: Whites' identification and misidentification of violent and nonviolent criminal suspects. *Media Psychology* 4:137–156.

Opportunity Agenda. 2012. *Social science literature review: Media representations and impact on the lives of black men and boys.* Available from http://opportunityagenda. org/ literature_review_media_representations_and_impact_lives_black_men_And_boys.

Pan, Z., and G. Kosicki. 1993. Framing analysis: An approach to news discourse. *Political Communication* 10(1):55–75.

Parker, R. L., and J. L. Moore. 2014. Black male college students: Their perspective of media and its stereotypical angle of "blackness and maleness." *Black History Bulletin* 77(1):10–15.

Peck, T. C., S. Seinfeld, S. M. Aglioti, and M. Slater. 2013. Putting yourself in the skin of a black avatar reduces implicit racial bias. *Consciousness and Cognition* 22(3):779–787.

Ramasubramanian, S. 2007. Media-based strategies to reduce racial stereotypes activated by news stories. *Journalism & Mass Communication Quarterly* 84(2):249–264.

Ramasubramanian, S. 2010. Television viewing, racial attitudes, and policy preferences: Exploring the role of social identity and intergroup emotions in influencing support for affirmative action. *Communication Monographs* 77(1):102–120.

Ramasubramanian, S. 2011. The impact of stereotypical versus counterstereotypical media exemplars on racial attitudes, causal attributions, and support for affirmative action. *Communication Research* 38(4):497–516.

Ramasubramanian, S. 2013. Intergroup contact, media exposure, and racial attitudes. *Journal of Intercultural Communication Research* 42(1):54–72.

Ramasubramanian, S. 2015. Using celebrity news stories to effectively reduce racial/ ethnic prejudice. *Journal of Social Issues* 71(1):123–138.

Scharrer, E., and S. Ramasubramanian. 2015. Intervening in the media's influence on stereotypes of race and ethnicity: The role of media literacy education. *Journal of Social Issues* 71(1):171–185.

Smith, A. 2013. *African Americans and technology use: A demographic portrait.* Washington, DC: Pew Research Center.

Stroman, C. A., B. Merritt, and P. Matabane. 1989. Twenty years after Kerner: The portrayal of African-Americans on prime-time television. *Howard Journal of Communications* 2:44–55.

Stuber, J., I. Meyer, and B. Link. 2008. Stigma, prejudice, discrimination and health. *Social Science & Medicine* 67(3):351–357.

Tan, A., Y. Fujioka, and G. Tan. 2000. Television use, stereotypes of African Americans and opinions on affirmative action: An affective model of policy reasoning. *Communication Monographs* 67(4):362–371.

Team, T. 2015. AT&T closes DirecTV acquisition: Reviewing the concessions and benefits. *Forbes*, July 27.

Terkildsen and Schnell. 1977. How media frames move public opinion: An analysis of the women's movement. *Political Research Quarterly* 50(4):879–900.

Turner, J. S. 2014. A longitudinal content analysis of gender and ethnicity portrayals on ESPN's SportsCenter from 1999 to 2009. *Communication and Sport* 2(4):303–327.

Wailoo, K. 2006. Stigma, race, and disease in 20th century America. *Lancet* 367:531–533.

Wilkes, R. E., and H. Valencia. 1989. Hispanics and blacks in television commercials. *Journal of Advertising* 18(1):19–25.

Williams, D. R., and R. Williams-Morris, R. 2000. Racism and mental health: The African American experience. *Ethnicity & Health* 5(3–4):243–268.

10

CHALLENGES AND PROMISE OF HEALTH EQUITY FOR NATIVE HAWAIIANS

Noreen Mokuau, DSW, Patrick H. DeLeon, PhD, MPH, JD, Joseph Keawe'aimoku Kaholokula, PhD, Sadé Soares, JoAnn U. Tsark, MPH, and Coti-Lynne Puamana Haia, JD

Health equity, the attainment of the highest level of health for all people, is yet to be realized for many populations in the United States. Health equity focuses on diseases and health care services, but is also broadly linked to social determinants, such as socioeconomic status, the physical environment, discrimination, and legislative policies. For one population, Native Hawaiians, the indigenous people of Hawai'i, the elusiveness of health equity is reflected in the excess burden of health and social disparities.

The experience of health disparities for this native population is even more troubling as Hawai'i, with its diverse multiethnic population, is reputed to be the "healthiest state in America" (United Health Foundation, 2014). This paper provides a perspective on health equity for Native Hawaiians by reviewing population characteristics, identifying prominent health and social disparities, presenting programs that show promise for health equity, and concluding with recommendations for the future.

POPULATION CHARACTERISTICS

Census

In 2010, 5.2 million people in the United States identified as American Indian and Alaska Native, representing nearly 2 percent of the nation's population (Norris et al., 2012). In that same year, 1.2 million people identified as Native Hawaiian and other Pacific Islander (NHPI), with the largest groups being Native Hawaiian (527,000), Samoan (184,000), and Chamorro or Guamanian (148,000) (Hixson et al., 2012). There were 156,000 people reporting Native

Hawaiian as their sole racial category and an additional 371,000 people reporting Native Hawaiian ancestry in combination with another race. Seventy percent of Native Hawaiians reported being multiracial with one or more other races. Although Native Hawaiians had the largest numeric increase (126,000) from 2000 to 2010 among all NHPI groups, they continue to grow at a slower rate than other NHPI groups. This slower growth, coupled with the rapid growth in other NHPI groups, caused the Native Hawaiian proportion of the overall NHPI population to decline from 46 percent in 2000 to 43 percent in 2010 (Hixson et al., 2012). More than one-half (55 percent) or roughly 290,000 Native Hawaiians live in Hawai'i, making up approximately 21 percent of the state's multiethnic population of 1.4 million. California and Washington hold the second and third highest Native Hawaiian populations, respectively (Hixson et al., 2012).

Historical Background

One cannot begin to understand the health inequities of the Native Hawaiian people without first having an awareness of their history. The arrival of Captain James Cook in Hawai'i in 1778 represented one of the earliest contacts of Native Hawaiians with the Western world. Within the first 100 years of Western contact, the Native Hawaiian people would experience a 90 percent decrease in population due to the introduction of new diseases, such as tuberculosis, measles, smallpox, and syphilis (Kana'iaupuni and Malone, 2006; McCubbin and Marsella, 2009). Western contact increased as missionaries and whaling ships arrived at the islands. These missionaries developed boarding schools, removed Hawaiian children from their native homes, and strictly enforced Christianity, English, and Western culture (McCubbin et al., 2008). The practice of Hawaiian language and culture would continue to be disdained as primitive and pagan. As nonnative contact increased, Native Hawaiians began to lose possession of their land, politics, and economy. Because of the decline in the Native Hawaiian population, foreign laborers were hired, during the mid-1800s, to work in the sugar and pineapple industries. These laborers (from China, Japan, Portugal, the Philippines, and Puerto Rico), along with missionaries and businessmen, eventually outnumbered the Native Hawaiians. The gradual loss of people, culture, and land culminated in 1893 with the forced removal of the Hawaiian queen by a U.S. military–backed group of businessmen and missionary descendants (Kana'iaupuni and Malone, 2006). Without a vote from the general citizenry and amid Native Hawaiian protest, Hawai'i became a territory of the United States in 1898 (McCubbin et al., 2008; Schamel and Schamel, 1999). It achieved statehood in 1959.

The U.S. government has made several attempts to make amends for the illegal overthrow of the Hawaiian monarchy. These included the 1921 Hawaiian Homes

Commission Act, the 1951 ceding of Hawaiian lands, and the 1993 formal apology to Native Hawaiians via Public Law 150 (*100th Anniversary of the Overthrow of the Hawaiian Kingdom*, Public Law 150, 103rd Congress, 107 Stat. 1510, 1993; McCubbin et al., 2008). Although these acts have not led to improved conditions for the Native Hawaiian people, they have contributed to revived interest in Native Hawaiian customs and the Native Hawaiian sovereignty movement. During the early 1970s, especially, Native Hawaiians gained a renewed interest and pride in their traditional culture and in improving their social conditions. Beginning with protests against land abuses, the exploitative conditions of Native Hawaiians, and claims to birthrights, the Native Hawaiian sovereignty movement evolved to include goals of self-government, the creation of a public education system in the Native Hawaiian language, and legal entitlements to a national land base, including water rights (Trask, 1999). Public Law 150 identified the 1893 overthrow of the Native Hawaiian government as "illegal," called for reconciliation between the United States and the Native Hawaiian people, and identified the resilience of the Native Hawaiian people to preserve their cultural identity. This resolution especially emboldened Native Hawaiian sovereignty supporters. In 2000 the Native Hawaiian Reorganization Bill, also known as the Akaka Bill, was introduced with the goal of initiating a process by which a Native Hawaiian governing entity would be recognized by the United States (U.S. Congress, Senate, Committee on Indian Affairs, 2005). Although several revisions to the bill have been made, it was voted down by the U.S. Senate. Today, many Native Hawaiians continue to call for self-determination and self-governance.

Impact of Historical and Cultural Losses on Health

The Native Hawaiian experience has often been likened to that of the Native American, especially when addressing the effects of historical events on the current health and overall well-being of these groups. Both groups have experienced a colonizing majority who has subjugated them to long-term injustice and discrimination (Duran and Walters, 2004). The terms historical or multigenerational trauma/loss describe the cumulative impact of this colonization, oppression, and cultural suppression that continue to impact these groups' quality of life (Kirmayer et al., 2014). Even President Clinton, in his 1993 apology to Native Hawaiians, noted the "devastating" effects that Hawai'i's historical experiences have left on its people (Public Law 150). These losses include the following: loss of their original agricultural and aquacultural way of life due to urbanization (Liu and Alameda, 2011), the replacement of the Hawaiian language with English in legal and educational settings (Liu and Alameda, 2011), limited access to Native foods due to cost and restricted land-use policies, and relegation of native culture to Western depictions of Polynesian culture for tourist advertisements (Kanaʻiaupuni and Malone, 2006). Although the overthrow of the Kingdom of Hawaiʻi occurred more than a century ago, historical loss of population, land, culture, and self-identity has shaped the economic and psychosocial landscapes of Hawaiʻi's people and limits their ability to actualize optimal health.

HEALTH DISPARITIES

The Native Hawaiian population experiences numerous social and health disparities. In Hawaiʻi, Native Hawaiians have the shortest life expectancy and exhibit higher mortality rates than the total population due to heart disease, cancer, stroke, and diabetes. Poor health is inextricably linked to socioeconomic factors, and Native Hawaiians are more likely to live below the poverty level, experience higher rates of unemployment, live in crowded and impoverished conditions, and experience imprisonment (Naya, 2007; OHA, 2010). Noteworthy and disturbing is the high percentage of Native Hawaiians who are homeless in their own island homeland (Yamane et al., 2010). As many Native Hawaiians hold a holistic view of health in which family, community, land, and spiritual realms are interrelated, the cultural trauma/loss that continues today greatly impacts this group and is manifested in their many health disparities. In context of the numerous health and social disparities confronting Native Hawaiians, we highlight a few disparities with significant impact.

Cardiovascular and Cerebrovascular Disease

Cardiovascular disease (CVD) includes coronary heart disease (CHD) and cerebrovascular disease resulting in stroke. CHD and stroke are the first- and third-leading causes of death for Native Hawaiians, respectively (Balabis et al., 2007). Compared to other ethnic groups in Hawaiʻi, the prevalence of CHD has increased over the past 4 years for Native Hawaiians (currently at 4.2 percent), which is twice that of European Americans and three times that of Japanese Americans. Similar trends are seen for stroke, the prevalence of which in Native Hawaiians has also been increasing to twice that among other ethnic groups in Hawaiʻi. Native Hawaiians are also afflicted by stroke an average of 10 years younger than others (Nakagawa et al., 2013). Hypertension and obesity are CHD and stroke risk factors and they are also disproportionately higher for Native Hawaiians (Nguyen and Salvail, 2013). Studies have linked the higher prevalence of hypertension and obesity to perceptions of racism in Native Hawaiians (Kaholokula et al., 2010; McCubbin and Antonio, 2012). Overall, Native Hawaiians have among the highest mortality rates due to CVD with rates 34 percent higher than the general population (Balabis et al., 2007).

Cancer

As with other populations, cancer is the second leading cause of death for Native Hawaiians. However, troubling variations in incidence and mortality rates for the leading cancer sites are observed for Native Hawaiians. In Hawai'i, when compared with the other major ethnic groups, the overall cancer incidence rates were highest for Native Hawaiian women, and overall cancer mortality rates were highest for both Native Hawaiian men and women (American Cancer Society, Cancer Research Center of Hawai'i, and Hawai'i Department of Health, 2010). The leading cause of cancer death for all populations is lung cancer, but in Hawai'i, it is highest for both Native Hawaiian men and women. Despite improvements in breast cancer prevention and treatment, Native Hawaiian women continue to have the highest incidence and mortality rates. The explanations for these disparities relate to external, internal, and lifestyle factors ('Imi Hale, 2015) and could include the lack of culturally appropriate interventions, late detection, diagnoses at more advanced stages, genetic markers of tumor aggressiveness, and high prevalence of tobacco use (Mokuau et al., 2012). Examples of culturally tailored interventions include home-based family education, a screening intervention in a church setting, and hospital-based, patient navigator programs ('Imi Hale, 2015; Ka'opua et al., 2011; Mokuau et al., 2012). The undeniable improvements in cancer diagnosis and care in the last several decades will need further refinement to effectively impact cancer disparities in the Native Hawaiian population.

Diabetes

The prevalence of diabetes when based on self-report of its diagnosis is twice that of European Americans (11.6 percent vs. 5.1 percent) and higher than among other ethnic groups and the general population (Nguyen and Salvail, 2013). When based on actual screening for diabetes, its prevalence for Native Hawaiians nearly doubles because just as many have the disease but are unaware as those who have been diagnosed, and the gap between them and European Americans widens fourfold (Grandinetti et al., 2007). Overall, the mortality rate due to diabetes in Native Hawaiians is twice that for the entire state of Hawai'i (Johnson et al., 2004). As noted earlier, the prevalence of obesity, a major risk factor for diabetes, is higher among Native Hawaiians than other ethnic groups.

Large within-group differences in the risk for diabetes among Native Hawaiians have been found in relation to acculturation modes. It has been theorized that people who undergo an acculturation process, whether voluntarily or involuntarily, eventually settle into a mode of acculturation to adapt to the demands of the dominant mainstream, and the mode they settle into can affect their mental and physical health status (Berry, 2003). They can settle into one of four acculturation modes: (1) an integrated mode in which they identify highly with both their traditional ethnic heritage and the dominant mainstream cultural group; (2) a separatist mode (retermed here as traditional mode) in which they identify highly only with their traditional ethnic heritage; (3) an assimilated mode in which they identify highly only with the dominant mainstream cultural group; or (4) a marginalized mode in which they do not strongly identify with either their traditional ethnic or the mainstream cultural group.

Seventy-seven percent of Native Hawaiians are found to be in an integrated mode, 17 percent in a traditional mode, 4 percent in a marginalized mode, and 2 percent in an assimilated mode (Kaholokula et al., 2008). When comparing across the two most frequent acculturation modes, the prevalence of diabetes is as high as 27.9 percent for Native Hawaiians in a traditional mode compared to 15.4 percent for Native Hawaiians in an integrated mode (Kaholokula et al., 2008). It is hypothesized that these acculturation modes are markers of the degree of psychosocial stressors (e.g., discrimination) and cultural discord (e.g., policies that restrict one from practicing his or her culture) differentially experienced by Native Hawaiians, which places some at a greater risk for diabetes than others (Kaholokula et al., 2009).

Substance Abuse

Substance abuse and dependence are prominent health concerns for Native Hawaiians. Rates of illicit drug use are among the highest for Native Hawaiians, with evidence that they are increasing. Among persons age 12 or older, illicit drug use for Native Hawaiians or other Pacific Islanders was 3.5 percent in 2013 and 5.2 percent in 2014, compared with national averages of 2.6 and 2.7 percent, respectively (SAMHSA, 2015). In 2014, the rate of substance abuse or dependence (illicit drugs or alcohol) was 10 percent for Native Hawaiians or other Pacific Islanders and 8.1 percent for the nation. Further, emerging information indicates that mixed-race groups, such as Native Hawaiians, are at greater risk for substance abuse (Wu et al., 2013). Substance abuse in the Native Hawaiian population is associated with an array of social and behavioral problems including higher rates of depression and suicide, unsafe sexual practices with multiple partners, increased violence in multiple settings, and a disproportionate burden from incarceration (Edwards et al., 2010; Nishimura et al., 2005; OHA, 2010). There are multiple and complex explanations for these disparities when compared to other populations, including higher social, environmental, and economic risk factors; poorer access to care; and inappropriate care (SAMHSA, 2015).

Aging

The United States is experiencing rapid growth in its older population with estimates suggesting that by 2030 more than 20 percent of the nation's residents will be age 65 years and older (Ortman et al., 2014). In Hawai'i, residents have the greatest longevity of all 50 states (Lewis and Burd-Sharps, 2014) and report the "highest well-being" for older adults in the nation (Gallup-Healthways, 2015). Yet, in harsh contrast, Native Hawaiians have the shortest life expectancy of the major ethnic groups in Hawai'i (Ka'opua et al., 2011). Native Hawaiian older adults experience disparities in heart disease, cancer, and diabetes and increasing problems with dementia and Alzheimer's disease. They tend to live with families, and, although there is family desire and interest to provide elder care, emerging issues of caregiver burnout and stress are increasingly being reported. Health and caregiving needs of older Native Hawaiians exceed the availability of services, but often the services available show low utilization. In a qualitative study using listening sessions, Native Hawaiian elders and their caregivers identified services of priority, including transportation, caregiver respite, and caregiver education (Browne et al., 2014). Caring for Native Hawaiian elders translates into supporting them aging at home and in their community, with sufficient resources to strengthen family centeredness.

PROMISE OF HEALTH EQUITY

When asked to describe important aspects of their health, Native Hawaiians described cultural knowledge and practice to be of main importance (McMullin, 2005). They believe that a balanced system that integrates all aspects of the self (biological, psychological, social, cognitive, and spiritual) with the world (individual, family, community, and environment) brings about optimal health (McMullin, 2005; Mokuau, 2011). Native Hawaiian cultural values and beliefs are organized around the collective relationships of the family, community, land, and spiritual realm. We present three examples of model programs in which these factors are integrated, enhancing their receptivity, acceptability, and relevance to the intended Hawaiian constituencies. These programs leverage pivotal legislation and policy (Papa Ola Lōkahi), demonstrate innovative research infrastructure to build indigenous research capacity (RMATRIX II), and implement progressive community-relevant interventions (PILI and HELA). With these model programs, there is the potential for health impact through policies that increase the Native Hawaiian workforce in health care, tailor research to specifically examine and treat health disparities among Native

Hawaiians, and develop new clinical interventions that are community based and culturally anchored.

Papa Ola Lōkahi

The landmark E Ola Mau: The Native Hawaiian Health Needs Study (ALU LIKE, Inc. 1985), the first comprehensive health assessment of the Native Hawaiian community, identified health status, needs, and concerns of Native Hawaiians and related them to historical and cultural frameworks. That study reported that Native Hawaiians have some of the poorest health indicators in the nation. In concert with these findings, the U.S. Congress enacted the Native Hawaiian Health Care Act of 1988 (Public Law 579, 100th Cong.), establishing Papa Ola Lōkahi (POL), a community-based/community-placed consortium to administer the act and "raise the health status of Native Hawaiians to the highest possible level." Three major initiatives are highlighted. The first was establishing five individual, community-based Native Hawaiian Health Care Systems (NHHCSs) that include Hui Mālama Ola Nā 'Ōiwi serving Hawai'i island, Hui No Ke Ola Pono (Maui island), Na Pu'uwai (Moloka'i and Lāna'i islands), Ho'ōla Lāhui Hawai'i (Kaua'i island), and Ke Ola Mamo (O'ahu island). The NHHCSs provide a range of health and social services reaching over 30,000 annually. The second initiative is the Native Hawaiian Health Scholarship Program, established to address the paucity of Native Hawaiian health professionals. Since 1991, over 250 Native Hawaiians have received scholarship awards to support education in almost 20 different primary and behavioral health care disciplines. More than 200 have been placed in the health care workforce in medically underserved communities in Hawai'i. The third initiative is POL's Native Hawaiian Health Master Plan which was first completed in 1989 and is periodically updated. The current Master Plan initiative, Ke Ala Mālamalama I Mauli Ola involves over 50 community and clinical partners, working across disciplines and sectors to update and achieve a shared vision on improving Native Hawaiian well-being and guide POL's role and responsibilities as the Native Hawaiian Board of Health (Akau et al., 1998; Papa Ola Lōkahi, 1998, 2015).

RMATRIX-II

Innovative research with its broad goal of creating new knowledge is essential in the commitment to eliminate health disparities among Native Hawaiians. RMATRIX-II (2014–2019)[1] is a research program funded by the National Institute on Minority Health and Health Disparities at the University of Hawai'i at Mānoa (UHM). RMATRIX-II is a continuation of a U54 clinical and translational research grant award begun in 2010 (as RMATRIX-I). The research program provides an infrastructure for research that improves island health, particularly among Native Hawaiians, Pacific Islanders, and Filipinos. The infrastructure is intended to deepen the relevance of health disparities research and consists of resources on biostatistics and health sciences data analytics, clinical research resources, regulatory knowledge, professional development, collaborations and partnerships, and community-based work. RMATRIX-II uniquely blends the senior leadership of the UHM John A. Burns School of Medicine with the Myron B. Thompson School of Social Work to provide a strong platform for interprofessional research in health. A major commitment of RMATRIX-II is to develop cross-disciplinary junior researchers in health disparities, especially those from underrepresented backgrounds. To date, diverse fields of study at UHM with a common goal of improving health have participated, including medicine, social work, nursing, public health, law, tropical agriculture and human resources, business, engineering, pharmacy, education, and Hawaiian knowledge. RMATRIX-II invests in research that responds to high-density Native Hawaiian communities such as Papakōlea, Waimānalo, and Wai`anae. Requisite to these communities are priority research areas of nutrition and metabolic health; growth, development and reproductive health; and aging and chronic disease prevention/management. Since its inception in 2010, RMATRIX-I and II have supported investigators who have produced over $25 million in contracts and grants, published over 150 articles, and presented at over 80 conferences in diverse areas of high need for Native Hawaiian communities, such as childhood obesity, teen pregnancy, diabetes, AIDS/HIV, dementia, heart disease, and cancer.

PILI and HELA

Several effective, community-based and culturally relevant health promotion programs have been developed for Native Hawaiians and other Pacific Islanders to address excess body weight and improve diabetes and hypertension self-care. For example, the community and academic researchers of the Partnership for Improving Lifestyle Intervention (PILI) 'Ohana Program[2] developed the PILI Lifestyle Program (PLP), a 9-month and 12-month healthy lifestyle intervention, and Partners in Care (PIC), a 3-month diabetes self-care intervention using community-based participatory research approaches. They were designed to be delivered by community peer educators in a group format across various types of community settings (e.g., community health centers as well as homestead communities). Both the PLP and PIC have been extensively tested via randomized controlled trials and found to lead to significant weight loss for Native Hawaiians with excess body weight (Kaholokula et al., 2013; Mau et al., 2010) and improvements in blood sugar levels for those with diabetes (Sinclair et al., 2013), respectively. The PLP was also found to improve both systolic and diastolic blood pressure.

The community and academic partners of the Hula Enhancing Lifestyle Adaptation (HELA) Project[3] designed a hypertension self-care program centered around hula, the traditional dance of Hawai'i (Look et al., 2012; Maskarinec et al.; 2014). This program is called Ola Hou i ka Hula (translates as "regaining life" through hula) and it was found to significantly reduce systolic blood pressure by 10.7 mmHg for Native Hawaiians with hypertension when compared to a comparable wait-list control (Kaholokula et al., 2015).

RECOMMENDATIONS

We have provided a perspective on the growing body of evidence documenting the health disparities among Native Hawaiians as well as the programs and interventions that show promise in the attainment of health equity. For Native Hawaiians to eventually achieve health equity, there are several interrelated requirements. First, there must be an institutional commitment by universities and, in particular, the University of Hawai'i, to train a sufficient number of Native Hawaiians in all disciplines to address health disparities and create health solutions. This quest was begun by the John A. Burns School of Medicine in the early 1970s with its special premedical school initiative and has now been embraced by the other health care disciplines, including nursing, social work, and public health. Second, there must be the establishment of culturally sensitive health care systems that will affirmatively seek out Native Hawaiian patients, as envisioned under the Accountable Care Organization (ACO) and Patient-Centered Medical Homes provisions of President Obama's Patient Protection and Affordable Care Act (Public Law 111–148, 124 Stat. 119, March 23, 2010). The Queen's Medical Center has historically played this role and, over time, several Native Hawaiian–administered organizations, such as Papa Ola Lōkahi (established in the late 1980s) and I Ola Lāhui, were established to provide culturally minded assessments and clinical interventions, as well as clinical training sites and/or scholarships for the next generation of Native Hawaiian providers. The latter program provides specialized, postdoctoral, psychological training expertise emphasizing the importance of integrating the psychosocial-cultural-behavioral elements of quality health care, especially for those with chronic conditions. Services that are culturally sensitive will include attention to dietary needs, community relationships, and cultural/spiritual values as well as the potential for the use of indigenous plants and herbs as medications. The neighbor islands of Hawai'i represent rural America with all of the traditional challenges of access, provider burnout, and insufficient specialty care; effectively using telehealth care will be necessary to address these issues (IOM, 2005).

Third, it is essential that there be a serious appreciation for the complexity of Native Hawaiian culture at the policy level, or it will be very difficult, if not impossible, to affirmatively impact the historical pattern of adverse health consequences. Further, one must reasonably expect that it will not be in the foreseeable future that our nation's provider-oriented approach to health care reimbursement will allocate sufficient financial resources for such a fundamental change in orientation, notwithstanding its importance. Native Hawaiian–administered programs represent a unique opportunity for the indigenous people of Hawai'i to control their own health care destiny. With the enactment of the Native Hawaiian Health Care and Education Acts, considerable federal funding has been made available over the past several decades for these purposes. Much of the federal financial support they receive is not directly tied to the specific amount of clinical services provided and is instead programmatic in nature, and thus can be the basis for necessary infrastructure support. Hopefully, over time, each of the programs will be successful in obtaining additional support from interested foundations, Medicaid, and private health insurance contracts.

The recent Native Hawaiian renaissance, as a direct result of the collective passion generated by the voyage of the Hōkūle'a, demonstrates the critical importance of culturally sensitive interventions. At the same time, it is important to appreciate that, although over the past four decades there have been more than 150 federal statutes recognizing Native Hawaiians, these are "stand-alone" in nature and rely almost exclusively on federal domestic discretionary funds for implementation. It is worth noting here that the Departments of the Interior and Justice have published a proposed rulemaking to establish a government-to-government relationship with the Native Hawaiian people in a fashion similar to that of Alaska Natives and Native Americans. In addition to this rulemaking, action at the local level continues to be heavily debated on the Na'i Aupuni process, in which Native Hawaiians are discussing government reorganization and sovereignty. Certainly one question facing any reorganized Native Hawaiian government will be the continued health care and well-being of its citizenry.

ENDNOTES

1. RCMI Multidisciplinary And Translational Research Infrastructure eXpansion (RMATRIX) is funded by the National Institute on Minority Health and Health Disparities, National Institutes of Health (2U54MD007584-04).

2. The PILI 'Ohana Program has been funded by the National Institute on Minority Health and Health Disparities (R24MD001660) and the National Cancer Institute (U54 CA153459) of the National Institutes of Health. Pili is also a Hawaiian word meaning "joining together" and 'ohana is Hawaiian for "family."

3. The HELA Project was also funded by NIMHD through RMATRIX-I (U54MD007584). Hela is also a Hawaiian word referring to a type of hula movement.

REFERENCES

ALU LIKE, Inc. 1985. E Ola Mau, Native Hawaiian Health Needs Study. Honolulu: Native Hawaiian Research Consortium.

Akau, M., W. Akutagawa, K. Birnie, M. L. Chang, E. Kinney, S. Nissanka, D. Peters, R. Sagum, D. Soares, and H. Spoehr. 1998. Ke Ala Ola Pono: The Native Hawaiian community's effort to heal itself. *Pacific Health Dialog* 5(2):232–238.

American Cancer Society, Cancer Research Center of Hawai'i, and Hawai'i Department of Health. 2010. *Hawai'i Cancer Facts & Figures 2010*. Honolulu: Authors. Available from http://www.uhcancercenter.org/pdf/hcff-pub-2010.pdf.

Balabis, J., A. Pobutsky, K. Kromer Baker, C. Tottori, and F. Salvail. 2007. *The burden of cardiovascular disease in Hawai'i 2007*. Honolulu: Hawai'i State Department of Health. Available from http://health.hawaii.gov/brfss/files/2013/11/TheBurdenofCVD.pdf.

Berry, J. W. 2003. Conceptual approaches to acculturation. In *Acculturation: Advances in theory, measurement and applied research*, edited by K. M. Chun, P. Balls-Organista, and G. Marin. Washington, DC: American Psychological Association. Pp. 17–37.

Browne, C. V., N. Mokuau, L. S. Ka'opua, B. J. Kim, P. Higuchi, and K. L. Braun. 2014. Listening to the voices of Native Hawaiian elders and 'ohana caregivers: Discussions on aging, health, and care preferences. *Journal of Cross Cultural Gerontology* 29:131–151.

Duran, B., and K. Walters. 2004. HIV/AIDS prevention in "Indian Country": Current practice, indigenist etiology models, and postcolonial approaches to change. *AIDS Education and Prevention* 16(3):187–201.

Edwards, C., D. Giroux, and S. Okamoto. 2010. A review of the literature on Native Hawaiian youth and drug use: Implications for research and practice. *Journal of Ethnicity in Substance Abuse* 9:153–172.

Gallup-Healthways. 2015. *State of American well-being: State well-being rankings for older Americans*. Available from http://www.well-beingindex.com/older-americans-report.

Grandinetti, A., J. K. Kaholokula, A. G. Theriault, J. M. Mor, H. K. Chang, and C. Waslien. 2007. Prevalence of diabetes and glucose intolerance in an ethnically diverse rural community of Hawai'i. *Ethnicity & Disease* 17(2):245–250.

Hixson, L., B. B. Hepler, and M. O. Kim. 2012. *Native Hawaiians and Other Pacific Islander population: 2010*. Washington, DC: U.S. Census Bureau.

'Imi Hale. 2015. Native Hawaiian cancer fact sheet. Available from http://www.imihale.org/pubs/brochures/Cancer%20Brochures/Cancer_Fact_Sheet.pdf.

IOM (Institute of Medicine). 2005. *Quality through collaboration: The future of rural health*. Washington, DC: The National Academies Press.

Johnson, D. B., N. Omaya, L. LeMarchand, and L. Wilkens. 2004. Native Hawaiians' mortality, morbidity, and lifestyle: Comparing data from 1982, 1990, and 2000. *Pacific Health Dialog* 11(2):120–130.

Kaholokula, J. K., A. H. Nacapoy, A. Grandinetti, and H. K. Chang. 2008. Association between acculturation modes and type 2 diabetes among Native Hawaiians. *Diabetes Care* 31(4):698–700.

Kaholokula, J. K., A. H. Nacapoy, and K. L. Dang. 2009. Social justice as a public health imperative for Kānaka Maoli. *AlterNative: An International Journal of Indigenous Peoples* 5(2):117–137.

Kaholokula, J. K., M. K. Iwane, and A. H. Nacapoy. 2010. Effects of perceived racism and acculturation on hypertension in Native Hawaiians. *Hawaii Medical Journal* 69(Suppl. 2):11–15.

Kaholokula, J. K., C. K. M. Townsend, A. Ige, K. A. Sinclair, M. K. Mau, A. Leake, D.-M. Palakiko, S. R. Yoshimura, P. Kekauoha, and C. Hughes. 2013. Socio-demographic, behavioral, and biological variables related to weight loss in Native Hawaiians and other Pacific Islanders. *Obesity* 21:E196–E203.

Kaholokula, J. K., M. Look, T. Mabellos, G. Zhang, M. de Silva, S. Yoshimura, C. Solatoris, T. Wills, T. B. Seto, and K. A. Sinclair. 2015. Cultural dance program improves hypertension management for Native Hawaiians and Pacific Islanders: A pilot randomized trial. *Journal of Racial and Ethnic Health Disparities*. doi:10.1007/s40615-015-0198-4.

Kanaʻiaupuni, S. M., and N. Malone. 2006. This land is my land: The role of place in Native Hawaiian identity. *Hūlili: Multidisciplinary Research on Hawaiian Well-Being* 3(1):281–307.

Kaʻopua, L. S., K. L. Braun, C. V. Browne, N. Mokuau, and C. B. Park. 2011. Why are Native Hawaiians underrepresented in Hawaiʻi's older adult population? *Journal of Aging Research* 2011:701232.

Kirmayer, L. J., J. P. Gone, and J. Moses. 2014. Rethinking historical trauma. *Journal of Transcultural Psychiatry* 51(3):299–319.

Lewis, K., and S. Burd-Sharps. 2014. *The measure of America* 2013–2014. New York: Social Science Research Council.

Liu, D., and C. K. Alameda. 2011. Social determinants of health for Native Hawaiian children and adolescents. *Hawaiʻi Medical Journal* 70:9–14.

Look, M. A., J. K. Kaholokula, A. F. Carvalho, T. Seto, and M. de Silva. 2012. Developing a culturally-based cardiac rehabilitation program: The HELA study. *Progress in Community Health Partnerships: Research, Education, and Action* 6(1):103–110.

Maskarinec, G. G., M. Look, K. Tolentino, M. Trask-Batti, T. Seto, M. de Silva, and J. K. Kaholokula. 2014. Patient perspectives on the Hula Empowering Lifestyle Adaptations (HELA) study: Benefits of dancing hula for cardiac rehabilitation. *Health Promotion Practice* 16(1):109–114.

Mau, M. K., J. K. Kaholokula, M. West, J. T. Efird, A. Leake, C. Rose, S. Yoshimura, P. Kekauoha, H. Gomes, and D. Palakiko. 2010. Translating diabetes prevention research into Native Hawaiian and Pacific Islander communities: The PILI ʻOhana Pilot Project. *Progress in Community Health Partnerships: Research, Education, and Action* 4(1):7–16.

McCubbin, L. D., and M. Antonio. 2012. Discrimination and obesity among Native Hawaiians. *Hawai'i Journal of Medicine and Public Health* 71(12):346–352.

McCubbin, L. D., and A. Marsella. 2009. Native Hawaiians and psychology: The cultural and historical context of indigenous ways of knowing. *Cultural Diversity and Ethnic Minority Psychology* 15(4):374–387.

McCubbin, L. D., M. E. Ishikawa, and H. I. McCubbin. 2008. The Kanaka Maoli: Native Hawaiians and their testimony of trauma and resilience. In *Ethnocultural perspectives on disaster and trauma: Foundations, issues, and applications*, edited by A. J. Marsella, J. L. Johnsons, P. Watson, and J. Gryczynski. New York: Springer. Pp. 271–298.

McMullin, J. 2005. The call to life: Revitalizing a healthy Hawaiian identity. *Social Science & Medicine* 61:809–820.

Mokuau, N. 2011. Culturally-based solutions to preserve the health of Native Hawaiians. *Journal of Ethnic & Cultural Diversity in Social Work* 20:98–113.

Mokuau, N., K. L. Braun, and E. Daniggelis. 2012. Building family capacity for Native Hawaiian women with breast cancer. *Health and Social Work* 37:216–224.

Nakagawa, K., M. A. Koenig, S. M. Asai, C. W. Chang, and T. B. Seto. 2013. Disparities among Asians and Native Hawaiians and Pacific Islanders with ischemic stroke. *Neurology* 80(9):839–843.

Naya, S. 2007. *Income distribution and poverty alleviation for the Native Hawaiian community.* Working Paper, Economic Series No. 91. Honolulu: East-West Center. Available from http://www.eastwestcenter.org/publications/income-distribution-and-poverty-alleviation-native-hawaiian-community.

Nguyen, D. H., and F. R. Salvail. 2013. The Hawai'i Behavioral Risk Factor Surveillance Survey, Hawai'i State Department of Health. Available from http://health.hawaii.gov/brfss/files/2015/04/HBRFSS_2013results_OCT06_Apr15.pdf.

Nishimura, S. T., D. A. Goebert, S. Ramisetty-Mikler, and R. Caetano. 2005. Adolescent alcohol use and suicide: Indicators among adolescents in Hawaii. *Cultural Diversity and Ethnic Minority Psychology* 11(4):309–320.

Norris, T., P. L. Vines, and E. M. Hoeffel. 2012. *Native American and Alaska Native population: 2010.* Washington, DC: U.S. Census Bureau.

OHA (Office of Hawaiian Affairs). 2010. *The disparate treatment of Native Hawaiians in the criminal justice system.* Honolulu: Author.

Ortman, J., V. Velkoff, and H. Hogan. 2014. *An aging nation: The older population in the United States.* Current Population Report P25-1140. Washington, DC: U.S. Census Bureau.

Papa Ola Lōkahi. 1998. *Ka 'Uhane Lōkahi, 1998 Native Hawaiian health and wellness summit and island 'Aha: Issues, trends and general recommendations.* Conference Report. Honolulu: Author.

Papa Ola Lōkahi. 2015. *Nana I Ka Pono Na Ma.* Pamphlet. Honolulu: Author.

SAMHSA (Substance Abuse and Mental Health Services Administration). 2015. *Racial and ethnic minority populations.* Available from http://www.samhsa.gov/specific-populations/racial-ethnic-minority.

Schamel, W., and C. E. Schamel. 1999. The 1897 petition against the annexation of Hawaii. *Social Education* 63(7):402–408.

Sinclair, K. A., E. K. Makahi, C. S. Solatorio, S. R. Yoshimura, C. K. M. Townsend, and J. K. Kaholokula. 2013. Outcomes from a diabetes self-management intervention for Native Hawaiians and Pacific Peoples: Partners in Care. *Annals of Behavioral Medicine* 45(1):24–32.

Trask, H. 1999. *From a native daughter: Colonialism and sovereignty in Hawai'i.* Honolulu: University of Hawaii Press.

United Health Foundation. 2014. *America's health rankings.* Available from http://www.americahealthrankings.org.

U.S. Congress, Senate, Committee on Indian Affairs. 2005. *To Express the Policy of the United States Regarding the United States Relationship with Native Hawaiians and to Provide a Process for the Recognition by the United States of the Native Hawaiian Governing Entity.* 109th Cong., 1st Sess. March 1.

Wu, L. T., D. G. Blazer, M. S. Swartz, B. Burchett, and K. T. Brady. 2013. Illicit and nonmedical drug use among Asian Americans, Native Hawaiians/Pacific Islanders, and mixed-race individuals. *Drug and Alcohol Dependence* 133(2):360–367.

Yamane, D. P., S. G. Oeser, and J. Omori. 2010. Health disparities in the Native Hawaiian homeless. *Hawai'i Medical Journal* 69:35–41.

ACKNOWLEDGMENTS

The authors would like to acknowledge Ms. Theresa Kreif, Assistant to the Dean, Myron B. Thompson School of Social Work, University of Hawai'i at Mānoa.

11

FETAL ALCOHOL SPECTRUM DISORDERS IN AFRICAN AMERICAN COMMUNITIES: CONTINUING THE QUEST FOR PREVENTION

Carl C. Bell, MD

For nearly 50 years, I have been trying to help children, boys and girls, who are in special education, foster care, and juvenile justice and who have difficulty learning, have been abused, and have explosive tempers along with poor judgment and poor people skills. I have been treading water in a sea of these children for years, so much so, seeing a child without these problems is like visiting a sunny island and being on dry land. Recently, it has become clear to me that many of the children I have been trying to help display behaviors consistent with a neuropsychiatric disorder the American Psychiatric Association is proposing to study by designating it as "Neurodevelopmental Disorder associated with Prenatal Alcohol Exposure" (APA, 2013). Since its scientific discovery in the United States in 1973 (Jones et al., 1973) and public health efforts by the Centers for Disease Control and Prevention, National Institute on Alcohol Abuse and Alcoholism, Substance Abuse and Mental Health Services Administration, and public health agencies, the knowledge that women should not drink during pregnancy is nearly ubiquitous. Unfortunately, too many women are drinking socially before they realize they are pregnant—nearly 50 percent of pregnancies are unplanned (Finer and Zolna, 2011)—only to heed the warning after they realize they are pregnant in a month or two. To understand how to address this public health issue, a little background in underserved population public health is necessary.

BACKGROUND

In 1967, African American physicians at Meharry Medical College in Nashville, Tennessee, were painfully aware of health disparities in the African American community. In turn, my medical training was entrenched in a public health and prevention model. The polio epidemic had provided a clear example of how prevention could eliminate health disparities, as the vaccine leveled the playing field between the haves and the have-nots. If one African American child presented with a rat bite, we were taught to treat the individual; if there were multiple such children, we were to treat the root cause, out in the community. We should get rid of the rats, or have our medical licenses revoked.

This concept of "getting rid of rats" has guided my career. In 1974, after completing a residency in psychiatry, I observed the common problem of African American children exposed to violence (Bell, 1987)—a potentially traumatic and preventable experience that I considered to be a "rat." Later, our work with Dr. David Satcher (the 16th Surgeon General, whom I knew from his presidency at Meharry Medical College) on his *Youth Violence* report (HHS, 2001) and the Institute of Medicine's *Reducing Suicide* report (IOM, 2002) highlighted the idea that there are protective factors in high-risk individuals and families that keep "risk factors from becoming predictive factors" (Griffin et al., 2011). Previously, several scientists (e.g., Garmezy et al., 1984; Luthar, 1991; Masten et al., 1988) had put forward the idea of resilience, but it had not yet received its due traction as a vital concept within the public health arena. In 2000, Dr. Satcher held his Children's Mental Health Conference (U.S. Public Health Service, 2000), in which he advised the nation's health care providers to focus on youth involved with child protective services, juvenile justice, and special education. These reports encouraged our public health systems to focus on strengthening protective factors, thus shifting our focus toward resiliency. After years of work, the issue of trauma, and resiliency in the face of trauma, has become an essential issue in public health—consider the impact our understanding of adverse childhood experiences has had on our nation (Felitti et al., 1998).

A STRONGER FOCUS ON PREVENTION
IN THE 21ST CENTURY

I continued to follow the prevention path set out for me, and had success in violence prevention, suicide prevention, and HIV prevention in the United States and abroad. Consequently, I was given the honor of participating in the National Research Council and Institute of Medicine's effort *Preventing Mental,*

Emotional, and Behavioral Disorders Among Young People: Progress and Possibilities (NRC/IOM, 2009). The Institute of Medicine's first prevention report (IOM, 1994) helped move the prevention agenda considerably. During the Clinton administration, a National Institute of Mental Health employee, Juan Ramos, first led this initiative. In a refreshingly nonpartisan manner, President Bush's administration continued to focus on prevention through its New Freedom Commission on Mental Health (2003). Thanks to the efforts of A. Kathryn Power (Director, Center for Mental Health Services at the Substance Abuse and Mental Health Services Administration [SAMHSA]), in 2004, the New England Coalition for Health Promotion and Disease Prevention held an important conference: "Evidence-Based Programs for the Promotion of Mental Health and Prevention of Mental Health and Substance Abuse Disorders." It was another stepping-stone to an even greater national focus on prevention. During the Bush administration, HHS supported the second National Research Council/Institute of Medicine prevention report (NRC/IOM, 2009), which provided the foundation for the Obama administration's strong focus on prevention within the Affordable Care Act. It was also this report that led to the first U.S. National Prevention and Health Promotion Strategy (National Prevention Council, 2011).

THE MISSING PIECE

Despite the resounding success of the 2009 NRC/IOM prevention report, it is now exceedingly clear that we had overlooked a major piece of the prevention dialogue: fetal alcohol exposure (FAE). Depending on when it is classified and who is classifying it, several diagnoses fall under the category of fetal alcohol spectrum disorders (Fasds), the overarching diagnosis that is caused by FAE. Within the spectrum, SAMHSA (2014) lists the following:

Fetal alcohol syndrome (FAS) is generally considered the most recognizable form of FASD. Individuals with this disorder exhibit the FAS facial phenotype, impaired growth, and cognitive and behavioral abnormalities (SAMHSA, 2014).

Partial FAS (pFAS) in individuals is characterized by FAS without growth deficiency but with most but not all of the facial features (SAMHSA, 2014).

Alcohol-related neurodevelopmental disorder (ARND) is a refinement by the Institute of Medicine to describe individuals with prenatal alcohol exposure and neurodevelopmental abnormalities, but no FAS facial phenotype. The neurodevelopmental abnormalities are characterized by a complex pattern of behavioral or cognitive conditions inconsistent with developmental level and not explained by genetic background or environment. Problems may include learning disabilities; school performance deficits; inadequate impulse control; social perceptual problems; language dysfunction; abstraction difficulties; mathematics deficiencies; and judgment, memory, and attention problems (SAMHSA, 2014). In a recent meta-analysis of 127 studies on diagnoses comorbid with FASD, Popova et al. (2016) found pooled comorbid prevalence rates of conduct disorder, and receptive and expressive language disorder at 90.7, 81.8, and 76.5 percent, respectively. Some diagnostic systems replace the term ARND with static encephalopathy/alcohol exposed (SE/AE) and neurobehavioral disorder/alcohol exposed (ND/AE) (SAMHSA, 2014). Of course, now DSM-5 has also proposed neurodevelopment disorder associated with prenatal alcohol exposure (ND-PAE) (APA, 2013) for this condition.

Neurobehavioral disorder/alcohol exposed (ND/AE) is used to describe individuals with prenatal alcohol exposure, moderate cognitive/behavioral impairment (equivalent to moderate ARND), and no FAS facial phenotype (SAMHSA, 2014).

Static encephalopathy/alcohol exposed (SE/AE) is used to describe individuals with prenatal alcohol exposure and severe cognitive/behavioral impairment (equivalent to severe ARND), but no FAS facial phenotype (SAMHSA, 2014).

The average layperson knows that when a woman is pregnant, she should not drink alcohol, because it has the potential to cause severe or subtle brain damage in the fetus. In turn, we generally associate FAE outcomes with newborns or young children. Moreover, FAE has long been considered an endemic problem within Native American communities (HHS, 2001). Although these medical and cultural rules of thumb may be accurate, the vast majority of workers in special education, child welfare, corrections, and mental health must now acknowledge how common and destructive this problem is for our nation as a whole. Like many clinicians, I have been seeing the impact of FAE for decades, but I did not know what I was seeing, nor did I understand its etiology. Additionally, all of the prevention efforts heretofore have brought health disparities and social determinants of health into the nation's awareness, but the lack of flourishing that is endemic to low-income African Americans has not yet risen into its consciousness. As you will see, the journey to reach the intersection of these varied issues was a protracted one; after all, how does a fish recognize water?

THE JOURNEY TO AWARENESS OF FETAL ALCOHOL SPECTRUM DISORDERS

In 1968, as a medical student, I researched the nutritional status of 50 low-income African American children at the Children and Youth Clinic in Tennessee (Bell,

1971). In the research, 8 percent of subjects had been born prematurely, but their age- and sex-adjusted weight/height and head circumference were within normal limits, based on the European American norms at that time. Eleven years later, Schutte (1980) developed a weight-and-height-distribution graph that was normed on middle-class African American children, and reassessing the 1968 sample reveals that a little more than 40 percent of the children studied had signs of impaired growth—a sign of FAS. In 1967, public health surveillance revealed that African Americans were born prematurely at a rate that was two- to threefold higher than among European Americans (Buck, 1967), and a disproportionately high percentage of patients that Meharry served were thought to have "sociocultural mental retardation" or "minimal brain dysfunction" (Nelson, 1966). I was puzzled at the root causes of these health disparities.

While working for the Chicago Board of Education in 1977, I again observed mild "mental retardation" and "minimal brain dysfunction" in their special education youth. By then, our understanding of child psychiatry had improved, and it was possible to arrive at a more refined classification of these children's symptoms. I categorized 274 children into 10 distinct categories: (1) organic brain syndrome/trainable mentally handicapped with explosive behavior, (2) educable mentally handicapped (EMH) with explosive behavior, (3) EMH with neurotic symptoms, (4) psychotic (autistic, childhood schizophrenia, adolescent schizophrenia), (5) borderline syndrome, (6) socially maladjusted behavior, (7) minimal brain dysfunction/learning disability with explosive and/or neurotic symptoms, (8) explosive behavior, (9) neurotic (anger/depressive) symptoms, and (10) psychophysiologic disorders. In retrospect, about two-thirds to three-quarters of these children exhibited multiple characteristics of FAE. This includes intellectual disability, speech and language difficulties, hyperactivity, high excitability, high distractibility with poor attention span, and poor frustration tolerance, all of which lead to poor impulse/affect control and can ultimately result in explosive or even violent behavior (Bell, 1979; Bell and Chimata, 2015). I wondered what was causing their affect dysregulation (Bell and McBride, 2010).

In 1996, the Institute of Medicine published its report *Fetal Alcohol Syndrome* (IOM, 1996), but I still had not connected the likelihood of the high prevalence of FASD cases in African American communities to their disproportionately high number of liquor stores (Altman et al., 1991; Hackbarth et al., 1995; LaVeist and Wallace, 2000). The previously mentioned association of FAE with Native Americans as well as with the pediatric population also impeded my ability to connect the dots. As such, the clinical actuality that FAS/FASD could persist into adulthood was simply not on my radar as a community psychiatrist. Moreover, I was oblivious to the fact that the overabundance of liquor stores in the African

American community could serve as a social determinant of health that produced an acquired biological disability of subtle brain damage. My judgment was
clouded: I did not recognize that this subtle brain damage could masquerade as
a whole host of educational, criminal, and psychiatric disorders.

For years, I continued to practice community psychiatry on Chicago's South
Side and consult with the Special Education Services of the Chicago Board of
Education, the Illinois Department of Children and Family Services, and the
Cook County Temporary Detention Center. I continued to see low-income
African American children, many of whom displayed what I considered an odd
cluster of symptoms: a peculiar form of ADHD; various learning disabilities;
intellectual disability; soft neurological signs; affect dysregulation mainly characterized by explosive, short-lived tempers; and naïve, childlike social interactions. Additionally, many of these patients had been victimized and/or exposed
to violence in childhood. At that time, I attributed these symptoms to the high
rates of prematurity (which I hypothesized could cause a subtle form of brain
damage at birth from intracerebral bleeding that preemies have that would persist
into childhood and adolescence) and/or exposure to violence, along with poor
parenting, but it still did not add up. Though I did not pin down FAE as a cul-
prit, I began to write extensively on the issue of children exposed to violence.
In a short period, through our and others' efforts, our nation became acutely
aware of this problem.

In 1985, as a member of the National Commission on Correctional Health
Care's survey team reviewing the entire Texas Department of Corrections'
(TDC) prisons, I learned from TDC that 20 percent of the approximately
20,000 mostly African American inmates had "mental retardation." It was clear
to me that something was going on in the African American community that
generated a large number of intellectually challenged individuals, and contrary
to prevailing theories of the genetic inferiority of African Americans (Thomas
and Sillen, 1972), I doubted that it was genetic inferiority. In later years, as the
nation's public health infrastructure was trying to fully crystallize its efforts on
prevention and resiliency, the criminal justice system was struggling with the
disproportionate number of African American youth and adults who were being
incarcerated.

The Children's Defense Fund (CDF), shepherded by Marion Wright Edelman,
began to take advantage of the increasing amount of information about the health
and well-being of the nation's African American citizens. There was a looming
question that was raised at the CDF's Black Community Crusade for Children
Juvenile and Family Court Judges' Leadership Council Fall Symposium in 2000:
"Why Are So Many African American Children Diagnosed with Attention

Deficit Hyperactivity Disorder?" By 2007, the CDF had congealed its focus on the early processes that caused so many African Americans to wind up in corrections, and a conference on promising approaches to end violence and strengthen communities in dismantling the cradle-to-prison pipeline was held at Howard University (September 25–26, 2007).

In 2009, a serendipitous consultation with the Temporary Juvenile Detention Center revealed that between two-thirds and three-fourths of the youth in the Cook County Temporary Juvenile Detention Center had problems with mild intellectual disability, speech and language disorders, ADHD, and specific learning disorders (Bell, 2015b). Accordingly, it was clear that something was still driving the problem of subtle brain damage in African Americans that had been evident over the years. The cradle-to-prison pipeline hypothesis was that African American children were being shaped and seasoned to become correctional inmates within their formative years. In addition, a 2011 random-sample chart audit on 20 percent (162) of the children in four Chicago public school clinics revealed that 39 percent also had possibly been exposed to alcohol when they were in utero (Bell, 2014). Biology and environment together influenced these children's early educational outcomes, which served as a driving force in their being slated for the juvenile justice system. The youth in the school clinics evidenced a palpable pattern in their medical records, progressing from diagnoses of ADHD, speech and language disorders, specific learning disorders, and intellectual disability (all possible indicators of being exposed to prenatal alcohol) to a diagnosis of conduct disorder. The latter diagnosis set them up for incarceration when their affect dysregulation led to behaviors that were interpreted as intentional, criminal activities, without any acknowledgment of the possibility that untreated and undiagnosed subtle brain damage was driving their behavior.

After nearly half a century of not "getting it," I was seeing a young African American woman who had been a ward of the Illinois Department of Children and Family Services (Illinois DCFS) and whose three children were currently wards of the State of Illinois. While I was evaluating her for whether she should be able to see her children and potentially regain custody, I noticed her extremely obvious epicanthal folds, flat midface, and strabismus. When I asked her why she had come, she not only a reported a history of ADHD, speech and language disorders, specific learning disorders, and intellectual disability, she also stated, "I have bipolar disorder, schizophrenia, and depression." When she was 8 years old, she had been given a diagnosis of bipolar disorder because she would have emotional outbursts related to frustration she felt within situations that she did not understand, for example while trying to learn reading or math. As a result, she had several psychiatric hospitalizations as a child and, despite her "mood swings" lasting only 30 minutes to an hour, she was placed on mood stabilizers; and despite their lack of efficacy in modulating her affect dysregulation, she was maintained on these medications for years. In addition, she began to "hear voices" in her late teens. Upon closer examination, these voices were coming from inside of her head; she referred to them as her conscience. These "voices" were clearly a manifestation of her "inner dialogue" or "inner voice" that every human being experiences within his/her mind. Because no one had bothered to get the details of what she "heard," she was thought to be schizophrenic and was accordingly placed on high doses of antipsychotic medications. When she was emancipated from the Illinois DCFS, she could not successfully adapt to life as a young adult and became "depressed"—she was assigned this diagnosis despite her obvious capacity for humor and her strong desire to do well in life.

Thanks to pediatrics training in medical school, it hit me like a ton of bricks—fetal alcohol exposure. Although I was certainly not taught to look for FAE in adolescents and adults or in psychiatric patients, I knew what I was looking at was that same picture. I quickly obtained a history of her mother being a teenager when she had the patient—poor women 18–24 years old have unintended pregnancy rates two to three times higher than the national average (Finer and Zolna, 2011). Her grandmother had told her that her mother had been drinking before she realized she was pregnant; but once she learned she was pregnant, the patient's mother stopped drinking.

The following week, I was consulting with the government of Manitoba, Canada (Healthy Living, Seniors and Consumer Affairs, 2012) on the work we had done for the Institute of Medicine's 2009 prevention report (NRC/IOM, 2009). I learned that 19 out of 20 youth in the Canadian detention centers had FASD (Popova et al., 2011). As an aside, this illustrated the principle that "culture protects" and the absence of culture places youth at risk. Individuals with intact cultural proscriptions are less likely to engage in risky behaviors such as drinking, unsafe sex, drug use, and so on, because their culture informs and guides them (Bell, 2011, 2013b). Because of this insight about FASD, *Clinical Psychiatry News* graciously published an Advisor's Viewpoint to inform the psychiatrists across the country about the problem of FASD that had been hiding within psychiatric populations (Bell, 2012a). In spring 2012, the correctional health care workforce was made aware of the problem of FASD in the inmates within the correctional system (Bell, 2012b). Again, part of the obfuscation in recognizing FASD stems from our basic medical training: We were taught to look for fetal alcohol facies in infants. However, FAE leads to so much more than our basic understanding of FAS or FASD; it causes children, adolescents, and adults to have difficulty with learning, controlling their affect, remembering important things, and adapting to social situations.

In September 2012, I was communicating with Dr. Renato D. Alarcon, MD, who was working diligently on the issue of cultural issues within the DSM-5 Personality Work Group, of which I was a member. At the time, I was developing my own criteria for diagnosing FASD in adolescents and adults who lacked the fetal alcohol facies, as I did not know that the American Psychiatric Association (APA) was considering a diagnosis of ND-PAE for DSM-5 (APA, 2013). In a communication regarding cultural issues as they related to personality diagnoses, I had raised the issue of FASD as a significant problem for African Americans. Although the intellectual and behavioral sequelae of FASD have been attributed to culture in African Americans (Nelson, 1966), the reality is that these behaviors are caused by the social determinants of health that put them at risk for subtle brain damage (Bell, 2016). With my new understanding of FAE, I underlined a significant concern about how DSM-5 would address this phenomenon that was largely due to social determinants of health, that is, the large number of liquor stores within African American ghettos. When the APA finally gave their work groups the completed DSM-5, I was heartened to see that neurobehavioral disorder associated with prenatal alcohol exposure matched my criteria exactly. There is nothing sweeter in science than the moment when two distinct processes lead to the same conclusion—the validation is unquestionable.

Although I was extremely late to the FASD dance, I felt strongly that this problem had been largely overlooked in the African American community. Science and advocacy were the only ways to bring light to this hidden epidemic, but the path was fraught with danger, as history has shown that attempts to address issues of African American public health have often backfired. Consider the efforts to address the issue of black-on-black violence (Bell and Jenkins, 1990). After Surgeon General Koop declared some forms of black-on-black violence a public health problem, several public health advocates successfully put this issue on the public health agenda. Shortly after this public health initiative, the problem was attributed to the drug trade, and the rates of incarceration soared within the United States (Bell, 2015a). Despite the danger, the 2010 publication of *The New Jim Crow* (Alexander, 2010) fueled the urgency to address the issue of FASD in corrections and society at large. We had to follow Albert Einstein's admonition, displayed outside of the National Academy of Sciences' Keck Building in Washington, DC: "The right to search for truth implies also a duty; one must not conceal any part of what one has recognized to be true."

Accordingly, proponents started to push the conversation. The National Center for Youth in Confinement was informed about the problem of FASD for the youth within their walls (Bell, 2013a). Abram and colleagues (2004) highlighted the high levels of comorbidity of attention deficit and hyperactivity disorder (ADHD) or behavioral disorders and affective, substance use, anxiety, ADHD, and behavioral disorders among juvenile detainees. In this vein, FASD was touted as a major cause of ADHD and behavioral disorders. It was hypothesized that the most common problems occurring in all youth—(1) speech and language disorders, (2) specific learning disorders, (3) ADHD, and (4) mild intellectual deficiency—possibly originated with FASD (IOM, 1996). Unfortunately, because confined individuals are a protected population, conducting research on these problems has been difficult.

In 2012, the State of Illinois halted funding for the organization that I had helped to build: the Community Mental Health Council, Inc., which took me out of leadership and the isolation from the wellspring of researchable ideas, that is, clinical service. I was forced back into direct service—the best thing that could have ever happened to me and the public health mission bestowed on me by Meharry Medical College. After all, our motto at Meharry was "Worship of God through Service to Mankind."

After some time on an inpatient psychiatric unit at St. Bernard Hospital in the heart of Englewood—one of the poorest African American communities in Chicago (Bell, 2014)—my work revealed that among 93 consecutively admitted patients, 32 percent met the DSM-5 "condition for further study," ND-PAE (APA, 2013). Around the same time, the National Academy of Sciences (NAS) Committee on Law and Justice decided to tackle the problem of harsh disciplinary practices within juvenile justice. The issue of FASD was briefly mentioned, but there is still a great deal more work to be done to document the high rates of FASD in juvenile justice facilities around the nation (NRC, 2013). In 2014, the Committee on Law and Justice also addressed causes and consequences of high rates of incarceration, but the issue of FASD in corrections did not make the cut, because there was not enough solid research in corrections to document this phenomenon (NRC, 2014).

Finally, during the 30th Annual Rosalynn Carter Symposium on Mental Health Policy in 2014, the findings from the research at Jackson Park Hospital's Family Practice Clinic came to the fore. In a family medicine clinic on Chicago's South Side, serving a population of 143,000 (96 percent African American with a median household income of $33,809), 297 of 611 (49 percent) of the adults and youth had neurodevelopmental disorders with 237 (39 percent) having clinical profiles consistent with ND-PAE (Bell and Chimata, 2015). Because of the Carter Center presentation, the January 2015 Newsletter to the National Association of County Behavioral Health and Developmental Disability Directors carried a front-page article on the prevalence of FAE in low-income African Americans (Bell, 2015c).

LATE TO THE FETAL ALCOHOL DANCE

Despite all of the progress in public health, there remains a glaring oversight: Since the late 1960s and early 1970s, the disorders associated with FAE were being observed in infants and children, but it was not fully clear how prevalent this problem was in society at large. There have been a great many luminaries who have been at the FASD dance long before I ever heard the music. They have come from SAMHSA-funded FASD centers of excellence: the Center for Behavioral Teratology, San Diego; the North Dakota Fetal Alcohol Syndrome Center; University of Minnesota, Child Psychiatry Department, Minneapolis; Center on Human Development and Disability, University of Washington, Seattle; Fetal Alcohol Spectrum Disorders Regional Training Center, Nashville, Tennessee; Centers for Disease Control and Prevention (CDC); and the National Organization of Fetal Alcohol Syndrome in the United States and the United Kingdom. They have been doing outstanding work. For example, Astley et al. (2002) documented that the rates of FASD in Washington State's foster care population were 10–15 per 1,000,[1] and the CDC even has an FASD app. In addition, neuroimaging of the effects PAE on the developing human brain is well established as strong science (Donald et al., 2015). However, considering the tremendous impact this problem has on public health, and although there has been some traction within the nation on this issue, there has not been nearly enough. Tragically, despite nearly 20 years of good FAE research, child welfare organizations, corrections, mental health, and special education are still not cognizant of its significance. Perhaps they have been deterred because they would not know what to do about it if they found it in the people whom they serve. Certainly, the proposed diagnosis in APA's DSM-5 of ND-PAE will strengthen the conversation, because there is now a label for what we have been seeing in juvenile justice, special education, child protective services, adult unemployment services, and adult corrections, among others, for years.

---

1 Although the CDC admits it does not know exactly how many people have FASD, it has studies that have identified 0.2 to 1.5 infants with FAS for every 1,000 live births in certain areas of the United States, and studies using in-person assessment of school-age children in several U.S. communities report FAS at 6–9 of 1,000 children (http://www.cdc.gov/ncbddd/fasd/data.html).

GATHERING MOMENTUM AND HEADING TOWARD A TIPPING POINT

Momentum is gathering. May and colleagues (2014) published a paper on the prevalence of FASD in a predominately European American, middle-class, midwestern city and illustrated that the prevalence of FASD was much higher than expected—as high as 5 percent in this population-based sample. Then, a wonderful thing happened that determined the size of the problems for children in child protective services. Chasnoff and colleagues (2014) published a paper on 547 children referred to their facility from the Illinois DCFS for behavior problems and observed that 28.5 percent had FASD, but had never been properly diagnosed. We discovered a FAE rate of 388 per 1,000 patients in a low-income family medicine clinic on Chicago's South Side (Bell and Chimata, 2015), and we suspect equally high rates in African American ghettos throughout the United States. Another recent paper by Rojmahamongkol and colleagues (2014) documented that pediatricians in New Haven County, Connecticut, were more able to diagnose Williams syndrome (estimated to occur at rates of 1 per 7,500) than they were able to diagnose FASD, which has been reported at rates of 2–388 per 1,000, depending on the population being studied (Bell and Chimata, 2015). Thus, it seems that interest in this issue is burgeoning. *However, there is not enough attention to this issue.*

WHAT NEEDS TO BE DONE?

The problem is now squarely before us. Consider the traction that the IOM received when it revisited the 1994 prevention report and published a second version in 2009. After all, there has been an explosion in prevention knowledge since 1994, and a similar explosion in FASD knowledge since 1996. Now, the provocative question is, "What needs to be done?"

First, NAS should convene a meeting of the experts to examine the current state of FASD knowledge. If there is sufficient new knowledge, NAS needs to develop a new report on FASD. It has been 21 years since the first FAS report from the Institute of Medicine (IOM, 1996). It needs to be revisited, but it appears that the correctional, child protective services, special education, and mental health fields are not aware of the breadth of available research and its importance to the nation's public health. I believe that we are at a pre-"tipping point" moment and it would help to finally give the attention to what the second NRC/IOM report failed to highlight—the issue of FAE.

Maybe the awareness of the problem of FASD is hampered by the lack of understanding about what can be done about it. I have seen this dynamic once before when I suggested that children be screened for witnessing violence. The response was, "What do we do with them once they are identified?" Fortunately, in terms of FASD, there are animal studies showing that, when rats are given alcohol during pregnancy, and are given choline while they are still pregnant, the damage done to their fetuses is reduced and their birth outcomes are better (Thomas et al., 2007). Unfortunately, I know of only one study, done on humans in Russia, that supports this strategy, but that study has not yet been published. Of course, this strategy would be easy to implement, as choline is an over-the-counter nutrient, and the daily requirement for this quasi vitamin has been well established and shown to be safe. Unfortunately, choline supplements are relatively difficult to obtain, as most drug stores do not carry them, and there are only small amounts present in prenatal vitamins.

There is some indication from animal research that giving animals with FASD choline, folate, omega-3, and vitamin A postnatally helps to correct the damage that alcohol does to the fetus (Ballard et al., 2012; Thomas et al., 2007). This might work for humans, as well. Unfortunately, there is very little choline in infant formula. If an infant is born prematurely or with low birth weight, it is bound to be choline deficient. The infant leaves the womb early, is usually fed formula, and does not get the benefit of the choline that is shunted through the mother's breast milk. In this vein, Wozniak and coworkers (2013) suggest that giving 2.5- to 5-year-old children choline postnatally can improve outcomes for children with FASD. Ross et al. (2016) has recently published exciting work on *CHRNA7*, the alpha-7 nicotinic acetylcholine receptor gene that has been shown to play a role in the etiology of ADHD and autism spectrum disorders, showing that its expression is positively altered by perinatal phosphatidylcholine supplementation.

It is fascinating how much animal research has been done with choline and other substances (e.g., thyroxin), but human clinical trials have been lagging behind. We must explore the reparative capacity of choline, and other supplements, both prenatally and postnatally. We need to confirm that this strategy is empirically sound if we want to have a true impact. Because the problem of FAE is so rampant in the community I serve, until the research pans out, there are some ideas for addressing the problems related to FAE. I have been suggesting that some patients take choline, folate, omega-3, and vitamin A and I have seen some positive results.

Of course, everyone is aware that women should not drink when they are pregnant—we get that. Nevertheless, admonishing women not to drink while they are pregnant only works if they know they are pregnant. The problem is that half of pregnancies are unplanned (Finer and Zolna, 2011): Most of the women I talked to, whose children have FASD, report that they did not know they were pregnant. Accordingly, primary prevention misses so many women who do not know they are pregnant. There could be an opportunity to intervene by screening pregnant women for mistakenly drinking in the first trimester and giving them high doses of choline, if it proves efficacious. For example, about 10 percent of women going into corrections are pregnant and probably represent a high-risk group. Why not screen them for drinking before they knew they were pregnant and give them high doses of choline? Of course, you could give all childbearing women prophylactic vitamins and omega-3; screen all recently pregnant females for a history of prenatal alcohol use; and, if such a history exists, give those vitamins and omega-3 to mitigate the effects of FAE. Such a plan would involve educating obstetricians about FAE and the potential benefits of choline supplementation. In this regard, their political voice could help put pressure on the Food and Drug Administration to add choline into prenatal vitamins. Fortunately, I have it on good authority that the obstetricians are starting to pay more attention to this public blight.

If the postnatal choline strategy works, we could do public service announcements to grandmothers who are caregiving for grandchildren who have learning disorders, intellectual disability, ADHD, speech and language disorders, explosive tempers, and who know that their daughters or daughters-in-law were drinking during pregnancy. Naturally, there could be collaboration with public schools to identify children in special education who have the characteristic histories of FAE, and a parallel conversation with juvenile detention centers and child welfare services. The identified children could be given choline, folate, and vitamin A. Of course, the possibilities are endless and, accordingly, it will take a diverse, multidisciplinary committee to flush them all out.

ONE SIMPLE CONCLUSION

Clearly, there is a great deal to be done regarding the huge problem of FAE. Without the leadership of the NAS and the National Academy of Medicine to create some synergy between all of the spaces where FAE shows up, I am afraid our nation will continue to flounder in this regard, and our public health will continue to suffer tremendously. By illustrating my own ignorance, I hope I have given others the courage to become aware and more involved in solving this national scourge.

REFERENCES

Abram, K. M., L. A. Teplin, D. R. Charles, S. L. Longworth, G. M. McClelland, and M. K. Kulcan. 2004. Posttraumatic stress disorder and trauma in youth in juvenile detention. *Archives of General Psychiatry* 61:403–410.

Alexander, M. 2010. *The new Jim Crow—mass incarceration in the age of colorblindness.* New York: New Press.

Altman, D. G., C. Schooler, and M. D. Basil. 1991. Alcohol and cigarette advertising on billboards. *Health Education Research* 6:487–490.

APA (American Psychiatric Association). 2013. *Diagnostic and statistical manual, 5th edition.* Washington, DC: Author.

Astley, S. J., J. Stachowiak, S. K. Clarren, and C. Clausen. 2002. Application of the fetal alcohol syndrome facial photographic screening tool in a foster care population. *Journal of Pediatrics* 141(5):712–717.

Ballard, M. S., M. Sun, and J. Ko. 2012. Vitamin A, folate, and choline as a possible preventive intervention to fetal alcohol syndrome. *Medical Hypotheses* 78: 489–493.

Bell, C. C. 1971. A social and nutritional survey on the population of the Children and Youth Center of Meharry College of north Nashville, TN. *Journal of the National Medical Association* 63(5):397–398.

Bell, C. C. 1979. Preventive psychiatry in the board of education. *Journal of the National Medical Association* 71(9):881–886.

Bell, C. C. 1987. Preventive strategies for dealing with violence among blacks. *Community Mental Health Journal* 23(3):217–228.

Bell, C. C. 2011. Trauma, culture, and resiliency. In *Resiliency in psychiatric clinical practice,* edited by S. Southwick, D. Charney, B. Litz, and M. Friedman. Cambridge, UK: Cambridge University Press. Pp. 176–188.

Bell, C. C. 2012a. Preventing fetal alcohol syndrome. *Clinical Psychiatry News* 40(5):8.

Bell, C. C. 2012b. An ethical conundrum in correctional health care. *Correct Care* 26(2):3–4.

Bell, C. C. 2013a. Common mental health problems experienced by youth in confinement—action steps. National Center for Youth in Confinement. Available from http://nc4yc.cloudaccess.net/list-all-resources/mental-health/192-common-mental-health-problems-experienced-by-youth-in-confinement-action-steps.html; http://nc4yc.cloudaccess.net/images/resources/nc4yc_mental_health.pdf.

Bell, C. C. 2013b. Culture: A key touchstone for treatment. *Clinical Psychiatry News* 41(2):10.

Bell, C. C. 2014. Fetal alcohol exposure among African Americans. *Psychiatric Services* 65(5):569.

Bell, C. C. 2015a. Gun violence, urban youth, and mental illness. In *Gun violence and mental illness,* edited by L. Gold and R. I. Simon. Washington, DC: American Psychiatric Press, Inc.

Bell, C. C. 2015b. Juveniles. In *Oxford textbook of correctional psychiatry,* edited by R. Trestman, K. Appelbaum, and J. Metzner. Oxford, England: Oxford University Press. Pp. 321–325.

Bell, C. C. 2015c. Prevalence of fetal alcohol exposure in low-income African Americans. National Association of County Behavioral Health and Developmental Disability Directors Newsletter. January 23.

Bell, C. C. 2016. High rates of neurobehavioral disorder associated with prenatal exposure to alcohol among African-Americans driven by the plethora of liquor stores in the community. *Journal of Family Medicine and Disease Prevention* 2(2):033.

Bell, C. C., and R. Chimata. 2015. Prevalence of neurodevelopmental disorders in low-income African Americans at a clinic on Chicago's South Side. *Psychiatric Services* 66(5):539–542.

Bell, C. C., and E. Jenkins. 1990. Prevention of black homicide. In *The state of black America—1990*, edited by J. Dewart. New York: National Urban League. Pp. 143–155.

Bell, C. C., and D. F. McBride. 2010. Affect regulation and the prevention of risky behaviors. *Journal of the American Medical Association* 304(5):565–566.

Buck, C. W. 1967. Prenatal and perinatal causes of early death and defect. In *Preventive medicine,* edited by D. W. Clark and B. MacMahon. Boston: Little, Brown and Company. Pp. 143–162.

Chasnoff, I. J., A. M. Wells, and L. King. 2014. Misdiagnosis and missed diagnoses in foster and adopted children with prenatal alcohol exposure. *Pediatrics* 135(2):264–270.

Donald, K. A., E. Eastman, F. M. Howells, C. Adnams, R. O. Riley, R. P. Woods, K. L. Narr, and D. J. Stein. 2015. Neuroimaging effects of prenatal alcohol exposure on the developing human brain: A magnetic resonance imaging review. *Acta Neuropsychiatrica* 17:1–19.

Felitti, V. J., R. F. Anda, D. Nordenberg, D. F. Williamson, A. M. Spitz, V. Edwards, M. P. Koss, and J. S. Marks. 1998. Relationship of childhood abuse and household dysfunction to many of the leading causes of death in adults. The Adverse Childhood Experiences (ACE) study. *American Journal of Preventive Medicine* 14:245–258.

Finer, L. B., and M. R. Zolna. 2011. Unintended pregnancy in the United States: Incidence and disparities, 2006. *Contraception* 84(5):478–485.

Garmezy, N., A. S. Masten, and A. Tellegen. 1984. The study of stress and competence in children: A building block for developmental psychopathology. *Child Development* 55(1):97–111.

Griffin, G., E. McEwen, B. H. Samuels, H. Suggs, J. L. Redd, and G. M. McClelland. 2011. Infusing protective factors for children in foster care. *Psychiatric Clinics of North America* 34(3):185–203.

Hackbarth, D. P., B. Silvestri, and W. Cosper. 1995. Tobacco and alcohol billboards in 50 Chicago neighborhoods: Market segmentation to sell dangerous products to the poor. *Journal of Public Health Policy* 16(2):213–230.

Healthy Living, Seniors and Consumer Affairs. 2012. *Rising to the challenge: A strategic plan for the mental health and well-being of Manitobans. Summary report of achievements: Year one.* Government of Manitoba, Canada. Available from http://www.gov.mb.ca/healthyliving/mh/docs/challenge_report_of_achievements.pdf.

HHS (Department of Health and Human Services). 2001. *Mental health: Culture, race, and ethnicity: A supplement to mental health: A report of the surgeon general.* Rockville, MD: Author.

IOM (Institute of Medicine). 1994. *Reducing risks for mental disorders: Frontiers for preventive intervention research,* edited by P. J. Mrazek and R. J. Haggerty. Washington, DC: National Academy Press.

IOM. 1996. *Fetal alcohol syndrome: Diagnosis, epidemiology, prevention, and treatment,* edited by K. Stratton, C. Howe, and F. C. Battaglia. Washington, DC: National Academy Press.

IOM. 2002. *Reducing suicide: A national imperative,* edited by S. K. Goldsmith, T. C. Pellmar, A. M. Kleinman, and W. E. Bunney. Washington, DC: The National Academies Press.

Jones, K. L., D. W. Smith, C. N. Ulleland, and A. P. Streissguth. 1973. Pattern of malformation in offspring of chronic alcoholic mothers. *Lancet* 301(7815):1267–1271.

LaVeist, T. A., and J. M. Wallace. 2000. Health risk and inequitable distribution of liquor stores in African American neighborhood. *Social Science and Medicine* 51:613–617.

Luthar, S. S. 1991. Vulnerability and resilience: A study of high-risk adolescents. *Child Development* 62:600–616.

Masten, A. S., N. Garmezy, A. Tellegen, D. S. Pellegrini, K. Larkin, and A. Larsen. 1988. Competence and stress in school children: The moderating effects of individual and family qualities. *Journal of Child Psychology and Psychiatry* 29:745–764.

May, P. A., A. Baete, J. Russo, A. J. Elliott, J. Blankenship, W. O. Kalberg, D. Buckley, M. Brooks, J. Hasken, O. Abdul-Rahman, M. P. Adam, L. K. Robinson, M. Manning, and E. Hoyme. 2014. Prevalence and characteristics of fetal alcohol spectrum disorders. *Pediatrics* 134:855–866.

National Prevention Council. 2011. *National Prevention Strategy.* Washington, DC: Department of Health and Human Services, Office of the Surgeon General.

Nelson, W. E., ed. 1966. Mental retardation. In *Textbook of pediatrics.* Philadelphia, PA: W.B. Saunders Co. P.1232–1243.

New Freedom Commission on Mental Health. 2003. *Achieving the promise: Transforming mental health care in America. Final report.* HHS Publ. No. SMA-03–3832. Rockville, MD.

NRC (National Research Council). 2013. *Reforming juvenile justice: A developmental approach,* edited by R. J. Bonnie, B. M. Chemers, and J. Schuck. Washington, DC: The National Academies Press.

NRC. 2014. *The growth of incarceration in the United States: Exploring causes and consequences.* Washington, DC: The National Academies Press.

NRC/IOM. 2009. *Preventing mental, emotional, and behavioral disorders among young people: Progress and possibilities,* edited by M. E. O'Connell, T. Boat, and K. E. Warner. Washington, DC: The National Academies Press.

Popova, S., S. Lange, D. Bekmuradov, A. Mihic, and J. Rehm. 2011. Fetal alcohol spectrum disorder prevalence estimates in correctional systems: A systematic literature review. *Canadian Journal of Public Health* 102(5):336–340.

Popova, S., S. Lange, K. Shield, A. Mihic, A. E. Chudley, R. A. S. Mukherjee, D. Bekmuradov, and J. Rehm. 2016. Comorbidity of fetal alcohol spectrum disorder: A systemic review and meta-analysis. *Lancet* 387:978–987.

Rojmahamongkol, P., A. Cheema-Hassan, and C. Weitzman. 2015. Do pediatricians recognize fetal alcohol spectrum disorders in children with developmental and behavioral problems? *Journal of Developmental and Behavioral Pediatrics* 36(3):197–202.

Ross, R. G., S. K. Hunter, L. Hoffman, L. McCarthy, B. M. Chambers, A. J. Law, S. Leonard, G. O. Zerbe, and R. Freedman. 2016. Perinatal phosphatidylcholine supplementation and early childhood behavior problems: Evidence for *CHRNA7* moderation. *American Journal of Psychiatry* 173(5):509–516.

SAMHSA (Substance Abuse and Mental Health Services Administration). 2014. *Addressing fetal alcohol spectrum disorders (FASD).* Treatment Improvement Protocol (TIP) Series 58. HHS Publ. No. (SMA) 13–4803.

Schutte, J. E. 1980. Growth standards for blacks: Current status. *Journal of the National Medical Association* 72(10):973–978.

Thomas, A., and S. Sillen. 1972. *Racism & psychiatry*. New York: Bruner Meisel U.

Thomas, J. D., J. S. Biane, K. A. O'Bryan, T. M. O'Neill, and H. D. Dominguez. 2007. Choline supplementation following third-trimester–equivalent alcohol exposure attenuates behavioral alterations in rats. *Behavioral Neuroscience* 121:120–130.

U.S. Public Health Service. 2000. Report of the Surgeon General's Conference on Children's Mental Health: A National Action Agenda. Washington, DC: Department of Health and Human Services.

Wozniak, J. R., A. J. Fuglestad, J. K. Eckerie, M. G. Kroupina, N. C. Miller, C. J. Boys, A. M. Brearley, B. A. Fink, H. L. Hoecker, S. H. Zeisel, and M. K. Gorgieff. 2013. Choline supplementation in children with fetal alcohol spectrum disorders has high feasibility and tolerability. *Nutrition Research* 33:897–904.

12

URGENT DISPATCH:
CALLING ON LEADERSHIP TO RESPOND TO
VIOLENCE IN BLACK NEIGHBORHOODS
AS A PUBLIC HEALTH CRISIS

Sharon Toomer and Raquel Mack, MS

Before our eyes, in plain sight and in real time, the people of the United States and all of its governing bodies, academic corridors, medical institutions, and public policy arena are witnessing the great human experiment that began in the 20th century and continues well into the 21st century: one group of citizenry is plagued with unceasing and prolonged violence.

That is the real-life state of affairs for people in black neighborhoods across the nation, and that there is no effective or targeted response to end the crisis is a commentary on the contemptible political, social, and economic failure of this nation to allow such conditions to exist for any of its own citizenry.

This failure to target and respond to a public health crisis and human atrocity happening in the nation's own backyard is a confounding and frustrating social and health injustice. What does it take for leadership in all sectors to aggressively and wholly step up and step in these impacted neighborhoods? Where is the immediate and targeted response? That is at the heart of this discussion paper.

The purpose of this chapter is not an academic, medical, or mental health examination of violence or the psychological impact of violence. Instead, our intent is to give voice to people who are suffering and overwhelmed with terrifying, life-changing, and life-ending conditions in neighborhoods across this nation as a result of the unrelenting and prolonged violence they live with day in and day out. We aim to message and appeal to the greater universe of expertise, leadership, and purse-string holders to respond to the urgent cries of the women, men, girls, and boys who are left to navigate and deal with the psychological aftermath of violent episodes. How can a people be expected to progress and excel or even exist under these conditions, when every aspect of their life—home, work, and learning—is affected by one act of violence?

For context and out of respect for those most affected by violence, we include perspectives of people who speak from firsthand knowledge or who, in their own experience with violence, offer invaluable insight. They are the voices on the ground that are too often ignored, rejected, or altogether dismissed by experts and leaders who stand on greater platforms of influence. The voices of the people most affected are vital to a comprehensive understanding of the conditions, what's at stake, and how to arrive at a solution.

But the overarching point of this perspective is to call attention to and present a case for why violence in black neighborhoods is a public health crisis that requires immediate, decisive, targeted, and swift action involving all sectors in a position to respond with expertise, leadership, and resources.

And, this, too, must be noted: the conspicuous absence of visible leadership and targeted response to the longstanding and progressively worsening crisis of violence in black neighborhoods is remarkable. Juxtaposed to the intervention in and response to the nation's opiate and heroin addiction public health crisis, the absence of visible and targeted leadership is all the more glaring.

LANGUAGE MATTERS: USE OF "BLACK PEOPLE" AND "NEIGHBORHOODS"

We use language that may not be customary for the primary reading audience. For instance, we use *black people* to describe the human beings we focus on and we use *neighborhood* in place of community. From our viewpoint, *black people* authentically and broadly describes and includes the people we highlight. The alternatives—African American, people of color, minorities, people of African descent—do not resonate with us in style, in content, or in this context.

In many neighborhoods, black people may be born in the United States and are generationally tied to this country, yet their ancestral and cultural linkage is to the West Indies, Caribbean, Africa, or Central and South America. The same is so for newly arrived immigrants of African descent. Brooklyn, New York, is an example of a borough (town) where the diversity of black people includes representation from across the world. All in all, news reports do not identify geographic lineage of black people, and crime statistics do not parse out ethnicity or cultural data when reporting violence in black neighborhoods. We want to recognize the diversity and nuance of cultures and we believe that is accomplished in the use of *black people* versus the alternatives.

Also necessary in this perspective is the distinction between *neighborhood* and *community*. These are *neighborhoods*, human and personal spaces, where black people live and violence is happening. *Community* is too broad a term that tends to detach the human element. This is an important language distinction because also missing in news coverage and crime statistics is the magnified shock wave of one act of violence on whole neighborhoods. One violent episode takes with it the primary victim and then it consumes all of the human beings in that neighborhood that are connected—directly or indirectly—to the primary victim.

Much like any other neighborhood, where lifelong and multigenerational relationships are formed, in these neighborhoods human lives are intertwined and bonds are cemented; often these relationships cross multiple generations. Also, many of these violence-plagued neighborhoods are located in densely populated cities where people become lastingly connected by way of shared home space in tenements or street blocks; schools; social activity; places of worship; base care and concern for one another; and, yes, hardship and tragedy. It is a culture of one hand washes the other and it is an essential way of life. Knowing other people's business is not always about being a nosy neighbor. Rather, it is a form of cultural communing. That culture is core to how people in black neighborhoods survive.

The people who make up these neighborhoods have dreams and aspirations and share in each other's life milestones, hardships, and upsets. These are living and breathing neighborhoods. The people who contribute to and navigate these neighborhoods are no less human and deserving of their nation's equal (to that of other citizenry) in measured intervention when crisis shows up and lingers.

We believe the distinction in language is vital.

DECISION TO FOCUS ON VIOLENCE IN BLACK NEIGHBORHOODS

Much thought and consideration was given to including Latinos in this paper. It is well documented that Latinos in U.S. neighborhoods are also dealing with an inordinate amount of violence resulting from street gang activity, domestic strife, and abuse of vulnerable immigrants. The intent here is not to minimize violence in Latino neighborhoods or any other for that matter. Rather than lump all groups into one issue we stand by our belief that all groups deserve a targeted approach and remedy. For those reasons we focus on black people in black neighborhoods.

TOLL OF TRAUMA

Ten years ago, on a Sunday morning in a Brooklyn, New York, apartment home, terror erupted when a 35-year-old man began shooting a firearm at family members inside the flat he shared with relatives (Jacobs, 2006). The night before, the man had celebrated his birthday and his liquor drinking had carried over to the next morning. The family matriarch and another woman had asked the man to stop drinking in front of the children. The alcohol-fueled rampage, witnesses speculated, might have been intensified by his failure to take prescribed medication for a head injury he had suffered. He "flipped out," said one witness.

Relatives and extended family members, including adults, teenagers, and children, were also in the apartment. What started as an ordinary festive gathering ended in an unimaginable outcome: the family matriarch, Mary Lee Clark, struck by several bullets, including one to the head while trying to shield her granddaughter, was placed on life support; several more children, adolescents, and adults in the apartment either witnessed the chaotic scene or were injured by gunshot; and a preschool-age child, Tajmere Clark, was dead. Bullets that struck her grandmother had also entered her body. It was the subject of the May 8, 2006 *New York Post* cover page.[1]

Tajmere was 3 years old. In one episode of violence, Tajmere's mother, Natasha Clark, was left childless and her mother remained comatose for years after. In that one act of violence, a family unit was indelibly marked and the tight-knit neighborhood lost treasured members representing two distinct generations.

In 2015, Dr. Rachel Yehuda, a professor of psychiatry and neuroscience and the director of the Traumatic Stress Studies Division at Mount Sinai School of Medicine, led a study showing the effects of trauma on generations. The team studied Holocaust survivors and their children's response to the trauma of the Holocaust. "Holocaust survivors responded to a horrendous environmental event," said Dr. Yehuda in a PBS interview. "In the second generation there is also a response to parental trauma [the Holocaust]."

Framing that medical research concept around the generational trauma experienced by black people and neighborhoods supports the case that an immediate

---

1   http://nypost.com/cover/post-covers-on-may-8th-2006.

and targeted public health response to violence is essential to the well-being and progress of those affected.

Complicated Grief Disorder

Severe and prolonged violence is the fixed condition for many black neighborhoods. This is common knowledge. There is a pile of evidence in the criminal justice system and in news media reports pointing to this static condition. In each and every episode of violence, without immediate and long-term care and treatment, it is hard to imagine how a family—much like 3-year-old Tajmere's family—emotionally and psychologically recovers from a traumatic event such as the violent loss of a relative; or how a neighborhood goes about the business of progressing through life productively and successfully when it endures unrelenting violence and loss of friends and extended family. And, equally hard to grasp is why they are essentially expected to recover on their own, without the vital health care intervention and support.

Take these explicit, yet weighty, questions into consideration:

How is a child expected to focus on school course work, test taking, social development, and overall learning while wrestling with a violent episode that he is not mentally equipped to deal with on his own?

How is a parent, relative, or extended family member expected to go to work, spend a full 8-plus-hour day focused on workload and being a productive employee, while also dealing with trauma of a violent act that took or changed the life of a loved one?

How are educators expected to not only teach course study, but also manage the unpredictable responses to violence visited on the students in their classroom?

What we know for certain is that violence causes trauma.

Exposure to violent death causes psychological trauma and can result in complicated grief disorder. Complicated grief involves extreme immobilization, pronounced psychotic ideation, and severe symptoms that persist over a long passage of time. This can also cause a breakdown in psychological functioning (Horwitz and Wakefield, 2007). Being in a state of shock, experiencing denial, avoidance of loss reminders, and dysfunctional or health-compromising behaviors are indicators of complicated grief (Ogrodniczuk et al., 2002). Consequently, black people are at a greater risk of developing complicated grief disorder. Individuals who are exposed to homicidal and traumatic loss are at a greater risk for developing complicated grief (van Denderen et al., 2015). Black people experience homicide more frequently than the majority population and have elevated grief symptoms in comparison (Williams et al., 2012).

In July 2012, 4-year-old Lloyd Morgan was with his mother watching a charity basketball tournament at a playground in his Bronx apartment complex (BBN Staff, 2012). During warm-weather months, this is a time-honored neighborhood gathering of friends, relatives, extended family, and neighbors. At the event, a teenager with a gun opened fire and missed his intended target. A bullet struck and killed Lloyd. This kind of violent scene has become a regular news story, but in this particular horror of violence, Lloyd's mother, Shianne Norman, showed in front of news cameras the emotional and psychological toll of trauma resulting from violence. It is a heart-wrenching, unfiltered communiqué from an anguished mother, and in her anguish-driven words to her son's killer, she gives the world a glimpse of the effects of violence:

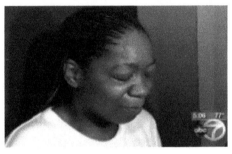

You destroyed me; you changed my whole life in an instant, and I don't know how I am supposed to go on. My son was 4 years old. He just turned four this May that just passed. He was going to school in September. He hasn't gotten to live his life yet. He hasn't gotten to do anything.[2]

Neighborhood Violence

Violence is prevalent in the metropolitan areas of many large states. For example, as of 2015 metropolitan areas consistently had a greater number of violent crimes than suburban areas (FBI Uniform Crime Report 2015[3]). There are multiple factors that are associated with a highest prevalence of metropolitan crime rates, including neighborhood disadvantage. Neighborhood disadvantages include high rates of poverty, joblessness, and residential mobility (Raghavan et al., 2006). The National Child Traumatic Stress Network defines community violence as exposure to intentional acts of interpersonal violence committed in public areas by individuals who are not intimately related to the victim.

---

2   Visit bit.ly/ShianneNorman to watch the video.

3   View the 2015 FBI Crime Report at https://ucr.fbi.gov/crime-in-the-u.s/2015/crime-in-the-u.s.-2015/tables/table-5.

Though gun violence dominates news reports, the legislative agenda, the criminal justice system and law enforcement narrative, elected representative outcry, and even the medical community's call for gun violence to be declared a public health crisis, firearms are not the singular method of violence in black neighborhoods. Undeniably, firearms are easily attainable and primary weapons of choice, but there is also sexual assault, use of other weapons in hand-to-hand fighting, and certainly the terrifying violence and harassment committed by law enforcement on black men and women (Noyes, 2014). There is no shortage of examples of community violence involving various methods of violence on black people.

Consider the following examples. In New York City, Glenn Wright, a 21-year-old college student helping his grandmother with chores was stabbed to death on a sidewalk by a group of boys, in a case of mistaken identity (Del Signore, 2012). In Chicago, Illinois, Derrion Albert, a 15-year-old high school student walking home from school, was beaten to death in front of many witnesses, including the person videotaping the killing (Khan, 2012). In Phoenix, Arizona, an 8-year-old girl was lured to a shed and brutally raped by a group of boys ranging in ages from 9 to 14 years old (CNN, 2009). In West Palm Beach, Florida, 12 teens kidnapped and held hostage a mother and her young son for hours, while they sodomized and raped her in one room and beat him in another room (Burdi and Diaz, 2007). In Richmond, California, a young girl attending her high school prom was gang-raped in front of witnesses outside of the school gym, where the prom took place (Netter, 2009).

Living under a stagnant cloud of community violence is traumatizing, and the immediate and long-term impacts of community violence are recognizable. Tony Herbert, a community advocate based in Brooklyn, New York, knows this too well.

Since 2003, Herbert has worked on the front lines of community violence. He has worked extensively with victims and families and publicly calls to attention the severe conditions people in black neighborhoods are living under. He is the go-to community advocate when violence disrupts a family and neighborhood. "Everybody is in survival mode," said Herbert in conversation for this perspective. "These kids suffer from PTSD." But, when there is a shooting, he said for instance, there isn't a team of counselors deployed to respond as when there is a mass shooting in a suburban school.

Herbert's observation is supported by research indicating the grim mental health effects of exposure to community violence, particularly on children and adolescents. Exposure to violence within the home and school can cause the development of aggression, internalizing, and externalizing symptoms in children and adolescents (Calvete and Orue, 2011; Reid Quiñones et al., 2011). In addition, there are racial and ethnic disparities in access to mental health services (Lê Cook et al., 2013). There are differences in the availability of mental health professionals in rural and urban areas.

These variations in geographic availability have been connected to the utilization of mental health services. In addition, black and Latino patients have a longer course of mental illness and a higher risk of disability from mental illness. Minorities are also more likely to be misdiagnosed with mental disorders. For example, black patients with an affective disorder are more likely than white patients to be diagnosed with schizophrenia. Additionally, Latino patients are more likely than white patients to be diagnosed with affective disorders (Primm et al., 2010).

Herbert also described an alarming reality for many children between ages 11 and 18. In his work with the nonprofit organization Youth Step USA, which uses the tradition of black sorority and fraternity stepping to provide a safe environment for youth, Herbert asks students at events how many have lost a loved one to violence. "Always three-fourths of the students raise their hand," he said. "At some events, there can be as many as 600 students."

Predator or Prey

In the early 1990s, at the age of 19, Alvin killed Mark, the neighborhood bully.

Alvin, who asked that his last name be withheld for privacy concerns, comes from a stable, working class family with decades-old roots in the Sheepshead Bay neighborhood of Brooklyn. Both of Alvin's parents were present in the home, where he and his two siblings lived. They were solid and engaged neighbors in the apartment development and deeply rooted in their church. Alvin, according to his mother, had started hanging out with the wrong crowd. It was a source of contention in their home. But, prior to killing Mark, he had not been in trouble with the law.

Mark was a couple of years older than Alvin and he, too, was rooted in the neighborhood. Mark, however, was infamously known to be especially brutal with violent force. His very presence instilled fear among his contemporaries and especially boys and teens. Rumors began circulating throughout the tight apartment development that Mark had it in for Alvin.

Though it may seem inconceivable that a rumor, on its own, could lead to a deadly outcome, Alvin explained the visceral reaction to being Mark's next target. He was overcome with the expectancy of terror. "The fear factor is what caused me to kill him [Mark]," said Alvin in an interview for this perspective.

"He was 6'4", 240 pounds and everybody was afraid of him. He was like a wild, savage animal."

Alvin was eventually prosecuted for manslaughter and sentenced to 7 to 12 years in an upstate New York maximum-security correctional facility. He served 12 years of the sentence before his parole. But, the gravity of what he had done affected him long after he killed Mark. In our conversation, Alvin articulated the process of understanding what it means to take the life of another human being. He was burdened. On his own, without counseling or therapy, Alvin exorcised what he had done. In that process he had come to learn more about Mark's tumultuous upbringing and life trajectory. Since the age of 7, Mark had been in and out of juvenile correctional facilities and lived a life weighed by familial instability, turmoil, and violence.

Likewise, but in a different way, a violent episode also consumes the people attached to the aggressor. Tony Herbert, who has witnessed the domino effect of acts of violence, explained how families of the aggressor become entangled and affected. "Families become victims, too. The embarrassment and being ostracized by the community you live in because your son is a killer. You didn't raise him right."

Herbert's point was underscored in a conversation with Alvin's mother Lorraine. She was 37 years old at the time and the violent episode took its toll on her and her family. She described the shock of the act itself and the fallout, which lasted throughout her son's criminal trial and into his 12-year prison sentence.[4]

"It was traumatizing. The helplessness, guilt behind what I did wrong as a mother. I felt so bad that my son took a life." Lorraine recalled Mark's name and thought about his family, his mother, and how living in her beloved neighborhood weighed on her. "I was depressed and full of shame and embarrassment." Out of fear, Lorraine and her husband made the difficult decision to break up the family unit and send their younger son to live down south with family. Their decision was a preemptive measure to prevent the path Alvin had taken.

That one violent act spiraled and rippled to impact every life it touched.

Alvin, in his own reflection, came to understand that Mark was a product of the environment he grew up in. "If you take a small child and expose them to constant violence, they will be violent. Either they will become predator or prey," he said.

This is how life plays out for black people in violence-plagued neighborhoods across the nation. This is their normal, even when that normal would not be accepted in any other neighborhood.

---

4   For the same reason as her son—privacy—Lorraine asked that her last name be withheld.

Alvin and Mark's path of violence is supported by research describing outcomes of proactive and reactive aggression. Exposure to violence has a direct influence on the development of aggression in youth and adolescents (Calvete and Orue, 2011). There are two types of aggressive acts: reactive and proactive. Reactive aggression can be defined as angry and impulsive outbursts in response to a stressor (Barker et al., 2006). Examples of reactive aggression include being violent to others when one feels fear or threat. Reactive aggression is linked to negative affect and is associated with increased levels of sadness, unhappiness, depression, and suicidal behavior (Fite et al., 2009a). Proactive aggression is unprovoked, goal oriented, and predatory. Reactive aggression is associated with behavior that responds to fear or threat of violence (Barker et al., 2006). Examples of proactive aggression include bullying and premeditated assault. Proactive aggression is associated with severe forms of antisocial behavior and psychopathic traits (Fite et al., 2009b). The etiology of aggression is extremely important because aggression is one of the best predictors for future social, psychological, behavioral, and academic problems.

Violence has an effect on the development of children whether it is witnessed or experienced. Research indicates that adolescents that have witnessed violence often exhibit fear and concern about being harmed and losing others (Reid Quiñones et al., 2011). In addition, community violence has a strong impact on the mental health outcomes of children and adolescents. A meta-analysis revealed that community violence has the strongest impact on posttraumatic stress disorder and externalizing behaviors, such as deviance and aggression, in adolescents (Fowler et al., 2009). Children exhibited greater internalizing symptoms, such as depressed mood and difficulty coping with stressors (Fowler et al., 2009).

These are the catastrophic and traumatizing conditions that people in black neighborhoods across the nation are living under. There is no shortage and, in fact, there is an abundance of evidence highlighting these conditions and the emotional and psychological consequences.

CAUSE OF VIOLENCE IN BLACK NEIGHBORHOODS

Over the course of more than a decade of working in the trenches of community violence, Tony Herbert, without hesitation, identifies economic oppression, existing in a constant state of survival mode, depression, and PTSD as the root causes of violence. "Violence is a symptom of those conditions."

Herbert's summarization is supported, in part, by statistics recently highlighted in a University of Illinois at Chicago's Great Cities Institute study (Great

Cities Institute, 2016). Results from this study show that 47 percent of 20- to 24-year-old black men in Chicago were unemployed in 2014 and not in school. Historically, and in broader context, the nation's economic, social, and political injustices on black communities, which are compounded by marginalization and institutional and systemic racism, are contributing factors to the crisis of violence and ensuing trauma.

Violence occurs in many different environments, including home, school, and the community. Mrug and colleagues (2008) researched the effects on adolescents of exposure to violence in different environments. The researchers investigated the difference between the development of internalizing symptoms, such as depression and anxiety, and externalizing symptoms, such as aggression and delinquency. The results of this study revealed that higher levels of violence exposure at home and school were associated with increased aggressive fantasies. In addition, higher levels of violence at home positively predicted delinquency and overt aggression (Mrug et al., 2008). Higher levels of violence exposure at school and home predicted more internalizing symptoms. Risk factors for developing internalizing symptoms included race/ethnicity, sex, and contributing family factors (Mrug et al., 2008). For example, females reported higher anxiety, African American ethnicity was associated with higher anxiety and depression, and parental use of inconsistent discipline predicted depressive symptoms (Mrug et al., 2008). Higher levels of anxiety and depression were also related to lower family income, greater parental use of harsh discipline strategies, higher levels of friends' delinquent behaviors, and lower school connectedness (Mrug et al., 2008). This study revealed that the environment in which violence is experienced can have a large effect on the trajectory of symptoms.

In September 2015, U.S. Senator Elizabeth Warren (D-MA) spoke before an audience at the Edward M. Kennedy Institute for the United States Senate. In an impassioned and precision-crafted speech, Senator Warren pinpointed a history of economic, social, and political barriers and excessive hardships that have done extraordinary and unparalleled damage to the black community as a whole (Warren, 2015). Her extensive and comprehensive understanding as an expert on the economy, law, history, and bread-and-butter issues positions Warren as a rare expert to tell the history and connect the dots on the social and economic conditions that plague black people, neighborhoods, and the community as a whole.

To this day, the conditions highlighted by Senator Warren continue, and until there is the political and societal will to comprehensively analyze, examine, address and, more urgently, remedy the factors leading to the present-day conditions, violence will continue to plague black neighborhoods across the nation.

In the meantime, while the great examination of *how* is left on the shelf, there is the urgency to address the trauma that stems from acts of violence in black neighborhoods.

"THE URGENCY OF NOW"—BOLD LEADERSHIP REQUIRED

The especially chilling rate and frequency of violence happening in black neighborhoods, and the unaddressed trauma that follows, is discriminate. The dilapidated environments that individuals are forced to live in are moderating factors to interpersonal violence. Neighborhoods with higher levels of social disorder increase women's exposure to community violence. Social disorder can be defined as "an array of threatening acts that occur between strangers within a particular neighborhood that can lower the quality of life" (Raghavan et al., 2006). These threatening acts can include violence, public intoxication, and drug sales.

Community violence is associated with increased rates of interpersonal violence (Raghavan et al., 2006). In public and private spaces, black people have shared a common belief that this sustained condition of violence would not reach the fever-pitch level in any other community or group in the United States without intervention and response. This belief is expressed in private homes, in barber and beauty shops, in places of worship, and even on social media. These are safe places where black people have traditionally communed and engaged in discussions that acutely affect them individually and collectively.

As it should be, war veterans, for example, receive targeted care (White House, 2016) and treatment for PTSD (National Center for PTSD, 2015). Domestic violence survivors are provided access to a network of resources to assist them, and there is an ongoing public policy campaign. In instances of mass school shootings, mental health counselors are deployed to support grieving and fear-ridden students (Office for Victims of Crime, 2015).

As a responsive measure to violence against women, then-Senator Joseph Biden (D-DE), in the 1990s, championed the Violence Against Women Act (VAWA), and in his role as vice president, VAWA was strengthened and updated in 2014.

In October 2015, as a response to the rise in white suburban and rural teenagers' addiction to prescription drugs and the illegal narcotic drug heroin, President Obama announced the White House initiative to coordinate efforts between federal, state, and local governments and the public and private sectors to address the public health and public safety crisis (Kuehn, 2014).

Following the 2012 massacre at Sandy Hook Elementary School in Newtown, Connecticut, the president, the U.S. Congress, and state and city leaders across the nation moved into action. President Obama even created a White House committee of top cabinet members, and assigned Vice President Biden to lead the group. In the border state of New York, Governor Andrew Cuomo, in less than

30 days after Sandy Hook, signed into law The New York Secure Ammunition and Firearms Enforcement Act of 2013, which is acclaimed as the toughest gun legislation in the nation.

In January 2016, President Obama moved boldly forward with executive action on gun control, yet the action is framed in response to and in the context of "mass shootings." Black neighborhoods are not dealing with mass shootings in schools, movie theaters, and shopping malls. It is white men and boys committing mass acts of violence. Black neighborhoods are dealing with individual (neighborhood) acts of violence.

The president, in his remarks to the public announcing his Gun Control Executive Order, referred to Dr. Martin Luther King's call for the "fierce urgency of now." Where is the fierce urgency of now in officially declaring violence in black neighborhoods a public health crisis and forging ahead aggressively with a targeted, multidisciplined, and significantly resourced course of action?

SOLUTIONS

So far, law enforcement, the criminal justice system, and more punitive measures through legislation (e.g., gun laws) have been the driving solution. But, those systems and measures have not curbed the violence and they do not address the emotional and mental health needs of traumatized people in black neighborhoods. "You can't arrest yourself out of the problem," said Tony Herbert. And to address the public health crisis, he said, "proper therapeutic programming is needed."

It is perplexing, given all there is to know about the crisis caused by extreme and prolonged violence in black neighborhoods, that there has not been urgent leadership to step up and mobilize responsive action targeting the critical health care needs of traumatized victims and survivors in black neighborhoods. A mobilized and concentrated action is needed, much like the coordinated effort to address the crisis involving suburban and rural teens, and the addiction to heroin and prescription drugs crisis.

The essential and immediate need is a declared public health crisis followed by targeted, multifaceted, and resourced action. What does that look like? For starters: visible, coordinated, and decisive leadership from all sectors and at the federal, state, and local government levels; a targeted strategy that homes in on black neighborhoods; and the unapologetic political will to boldly and publicly call this what it is: a public health crisis and social justice inequity.

In a nation of extraordinary abilities, intellectual minds, innovation, and abundance of resources, the United States and its leadership in the political, academic, medical, policy, and philanthropic spheres could one day be judged harshly on their failure to aggressively target and address the causes and traumatic outcomes of prolonged and sustained violence in black neighborhoods.

This is not a solution founded in idealism, nor is it the imagination of a utopian society. This is the rational and logical expectation of what leadership is required to do in a crisis. Nor is this a crisis for black people and neighborhoods without resources to solely own and figure out.

Economically, socially, politically, and culturally, black people and neighborhoods are as much a part of the United States as any other group of human beings or special interests. They contribute to the economy and are a tax base; serve in the military and send sons, daughters, husbands, and wives to fight in wars; show up loyally to a political party; and they produce and deepen the cultural fabric of this nation. Yet, black men, women, and children in violence-plagued neighborhoods across this nation are expected to live, survive, and progress under the most violent conditions, unlike any other group of Americans. In plainer terms, the urgent matter of violence in black neighborhoods is a U.S. crisis.

REFERENCES

Barker, E. D., R. E. Tremblay, D. S. Nagin, F. Vitaro, and R. Lacourse. 2006. Development of male proactive and reactive physical aggression during adolescence *Journal of Child Psychology and Psychiatry* 47(8):783–790.

BBN Staff. 2012. The impact of violence: The raw, unfiltered emotion of a mother in agony. Black and Brown News. July 23, p. 1. http://blackandbrownnews.com/nyc-tri-state/the-impact-of-violence-the-raw-unfiltered-emotion-of-a-mother-in-agony/.

Burdi, J., and M. Diaz. 2007. Teens ordered held without bond in Dunbar Village rape case. *Sun Sentinel*, July 18. Available from http://www.sun-sentinel.com/local/palm-beach/sfl-0719dunbarrape-story.html.

Calvete, E., and I. Orue. 2011. The impact of violence exposure on aggressive behavior through social information processing in adolescents. *American Journal of Orthopsychiatry* 81(1):38–50.

CNN. 2009. Rape victim's parents charged with abuse. Available from http://www.cnn.com/2009/CRIME/11/21/arizona.abuse.arrests/index.html?eref=onion.

Del Signore, J. 2012. The Lower East Side mistaken identity murder: Devastated family still waits for justice. *Gothamist News*. Available from http://gothamist.com/2012/03/12/the_lower_east_side_mistaken_identi.php.

Fite, P. J., A. Raine, M. Stouthamer-Loeber, R. Loeber, and D. A. Pardini. 2009a. Reactive and proactive aggression in adolescent males: Examining differential outcomes 10 years later in early adulthood. *Criminal Justice and Behavior* 37(2):141–157.

Fite, P. J., L. Stoppelbein, and L. Greening. 2009b. Proactive and reactive aggression in a child psychiatric inpatient population. *Journal of Clinical Child & Adolescent Psychology* 38:199–205.

Fowler, P. J., C. J. Tompsett, J. M. Braciszewski, A. J. Jacques-Tiura, and B. B. Baltes. 2009. Community violence: A meta-analysis on the effect of exposure and mental health outcomes of children and adolescents. *Development and Psychopathology* 21:227–259.

Great Cities Institute. 2016. *Young, black, and out of work*. Chicago: University of Illinois. Available from https://greatcities.uic.edu/2016/01/25/young-black-and-out-of-work/.

Horwitz, A. V., and J. C. Wakefield. 2007. *The loss of sadness: How psychiatry transformed normal sorrow into depressive disorder*. New York: Oxford University Press.

Jacobs, A. 2006. Girl is killed at a party in Brooklyn. *New York Times*, May 8. Available from http://www.nytimes.com/2006/05/08/nyregion/08shoot.html?_r=0.

Khan, A. 2012. Derrion Albert: The death that riled the nation. PBS *Frontline* report. Available from http://www.pbs.org/wgbh/frontline/article/derrion-albert-the-death-that-riled-the-nation/.

Kuehn, B. M. 2014. Driven by prescription drug abuse, heroin use increases among suburban and rural whites. *Journal of the American Medical Association* 312:118–119.

Lê Cook, B., T. Doksum, C. N. Chen, A. Carle, and M. Alegría. 2013. The role of provider supply and organization in reducing racial/ethnic disparities in mental health care in the U.S. *Social Science & Medicine* 84:102–109.

Mrug, S., P. S. Loosier, and M. Windle. 2008. Violence exposure across multiple contexts: Individual and joint effects on adjustment. *American Journal of Orthopsychiatry* 78(1):70–84.

National Center for PTSD. 2015. *Help for veterans with PTSD*. Department of Veterans Affairs. Available from http://www.ptsd.va.gov/public/PTSD-overview/reintegration/help-for-veterans-with-ptsd.asp.

Netter, S. 2009. No one called cops during gang rape, but some took pictures. *ABC News*, Oct. 27. Available from http://abcnews.go.com/WN/high-school-gang-rape-stuns-california-community/story?id=8925672.

Noyes, D. 2014. How criminals get guns. PBS *Frontline* report. Available from https://www.pbs.org/wgbh/pages/frontline/shows/guns/procon/guns.html.

Office for Victims of Crime. 2015. *Helping victims of mass violence and terrorism*. Available from http://www.ovc.gov/pubs/mvt-toolkit/victim-assistance.html.

Ogrodniczuk, J. S., W. E. Piper, A. S. Joyce, M. McCallum, and J. S. Rosie. 2002. Social support as a predictor of response to group therapy for complicated grief. *Psychiatry* 65:346–357.

Primm, A. B., M. J. Vasquez, Mays, R., D. Sammons-Posey, L. McKnight-Eily, L. Presley-Cantrell, L. C. McGuire, D. P. Chapman, and G. S. Perry. 2010. The role of public health in addressing racial and ethnic disparities in mental health and mental illness. *Preventing Chronic Disease* 7(1):A20.

Raghavan, C., A. Mennerich, E. Sexton, and S. E. James. 2006. Community violence and its direct, indirect, and mediating effects on intimate partner violence. *Violence Against Women* 12:1132–1149.

Reid Quiñones, K., W. Kliewer, B. J. Shields, K. Goodman, M. H. Ray, and E. Wheat. 2011. Cognitive, affective, and behavioral responses to witnessed versus experienced violence. *American Journal of Orthopsychiatry* 81:51–60.

van Denderen, M., J. de Keijser, M. Kleen, and P. A. Boelen. 2015. Psychopathology among homicidally bereaved individuals: A systematic review. *Trauma, Violence, & Abuse* 16(1):70–80.

Warren, E. 2015. Getting to the point with Senator Elizabeth Warren. Speech at the Edward M. Kennedy Institute for the United States Senate. Available from https://www.emkinstitute.org/resources/senatorwarren2015.

White House. 2016. *Joining forces.* Available from https://www.whitehouse.gov/joiningforces.

Williams, J. L., L. A. Burke, M. E. McDevitt-Murphy, and R. A. Neimeyer. 2012. Responses to loss and health functioning among homicidally bereaved African Americans. *Journal of Loss and Trauma* 17:358–375.

APPENDIX A: PAPER ABSTRACTS

FOREWORD

SOCIAL AND STRUCTURAL DETERMINANTS OF HEALTH AND HEALTH EQUITY

Authors: James Marks, MD, MPH, Helene Gayle, MD, MPH, and Dwayne Proctor, PhD

The National Academy of Medicine (NAM) serves as a national leader and advisor on issues relating to the science and practice of medicine, health care, and good health and well-being. This leadership also extends to the arena of health equity and social determinants of health. The NAM's Culture of Health Program, in partnership with the Robert Wood Johnson Foundation, recently released the consensus study Communities in Action: Pathways to Health Equity, which reviewed the science of inequity and highlighted nine communities taking action to reduce health disparities across the country. The program held its first stakeholder meeting in January 2017, bringing together leaders from a variety of fields, including policy, research, philanthropy, and community organizations, to reflect that interdisciplinary solutions are critical to furthering health equity in the United States.

Inequities in health have existed among humans since our beginnings as a civilization. In the mid-1800s, John Snow's discovery that cholera deaths were associated with a contaminated water pump in urban London catalyzed the formation of public health as a scientific discipline and cemented the significance of health equity in public health practice. As William Foege, former president of the American Public Health Association, once said, "The philosophy of public health is social justice." Because discrimination, poverty, and other forms of socioeconomic inequality lead to negative health outcomes in systemic ways, the goal of creating a culture of health must be central to the medical community's vision of optimal health for all.

Social determinants of health are the myriad ways community characteristics affect health equity, such as demographic factors, income levels, educational institutions, transportation infrastructure, and access to social services. The NAM's report and meeting repeatedly emphasized the importance of investing in early childhood programs and developing human capital for children; effectively using changing trends in communication and technological advancement to reach wider audiences; infusing health equity into every aspect of community living, from urban planning to economic development; and the importance of data collection in measuring and achieving health outcomes. The NAM's discussions highlighted the success of multisectoral approaches to better health and well-being, integrating efforts across community governments and institutions in health, education, law enforcement, and other social agencies to achieve collective impact.

Despite our scientific and technological innovation, the United States has been unable to translate these advances into better health outcomes compared to other countries. At this watershed time in our nation's history, every institution has a part to play in our mission of building a culture of health. The core value of medicine is the application of science to help those in need, and through community-based, multisectoral initiatives, we can live up to this idea and achieve health equity in America.

HEALTH INEQUITIES, SOCIAL DETERMINANTS, AND INTERSECTIONALITY

AUTHOR: NANCY LÓPEZ, PhD, AND VIVIAN L. GADSDEN, EdD

There is growing evidence to suggest that health disparities do not exist in isolation but are part of a reciprocal and complex web of problems associated with inequality and inequity in education, housing, and employment. Problems in health disrupt the human developmental process; they undermine the quality of life and opportunities for children and families, particularly those exposed to vulnerable circumstances. Health prevention and successful interventions depend not simply on the existence of care but also on access to care, quality of care, experience with care, and overall well-being.

A commitment to developing an intersectionality lens can advance health disparities research, practice, and leadership. Intersectionality is an intentional focus on the simultaneity of race/racism, gender/sexism, class/classism, sexual orientation/heterosexism, and physical disability by linking individual, institutional, and structural levels in a given sociohistorical context. The potential power of intersectionality as a transformational paradigm lies in two domains relevant to understanding social determinants. First, it examines closely and raises questions about the meaning and relationship between different social categories. It also pushes against the idea of "blaming the victim"—the simplicity of explaining health or educational outcomes through attributions to individuals' genetics and social behaviors alone. Second, by focusing on the convergence of experiences in context, it serves as an anchor in advancing social justice aims for all marginalized communities that have experienced and continue to experience structured inequalities.

Research has uncovered several interconnections between health and environmental and social factors but has not always shifted paradigms sufficiently to either disentangle interlocking issues or tease apart the ways social factors and institutional barriers at once interlock to prevent meaningful and sustainable change. Even the most agentive individual who is faced with daily problems of racial, class, gender, or disability discrimination may find fighting against these inequalities daunting. The relationship between oppression and privilege has become so intrinsic to societal practices that those who enact either or both may be unaware of their effects on others.

Intersectionality also acknowledges the ways policies and practices reinscribe positions of power, dominance, and oppression that contribute to the social determinants of health, education, and well-being. Social determinants are tied to matters of equity—to the availability and distribution of resources and power. These policies and practices are historical factors that reify inequalities, making them appear to be naturally occurring rather than the result of a social system.

An intersectionality lens can address the multiplicity of identities contributing to the social determinants of health for diverse populations of children, youth, and families and to move closer to effecting change.

IDENTIFYING AND IMPLEMENTING OPPORTUNITIES TO REALIZE HEALTH EQUITY THROUGH A LIFESPAN LENS OF LEGAL AND POLICY RESEARCH

AUTHORS: PATRICK H. TOLAN, PHD, VELMA MCBRIDE MURRY, PHD, ANGELA DIAZ, MD, PHD, MPH, AND ROBERT SEIDEL, MLA

The notion that health equity is a fundamental form of justice emanating from basic human rights suggests that health disparities should be central to health research, evaluation, and policy. In order to realize health equity, researchers must take a lifespan perspective and evaluate the policies and regulations that sustain health disparities. There is a need to move beyond the repetitive documentation of the existence of disparities, to a paradigm that illuminates the mechanisms through which health equity can be realized.

Health disparities refer to systematic health differences related to group membership and access to resources that are avoidable or malleable, and are primarily socially determined. The very definition of health disparities proposes that systematic differences between groups can be affected or eliminated because they are representative of social and politically based inequities.

Using a framework where health equity is central when prioritizing a national scientific agenda has the potential to reduce health disparities. Having more detailed information about the actual mechanisms through which disparities in susceptibility to disease are linked to access to resources, treatment quality and availability, and life-course trajectories is critical for recognizing the extent of the inequity. A distinct advantage of the life-course framework in explaining the systematic variations in individual and group health trajectories is that it allows for greater understanding of where equity is being realized or promoted, and where opportunities exist to overcome or undercut inequity promoting influences.

To raise the visibility of health equity as a matter of justice and ensure that all social groups have equal opportunity to reach their full potential as healthy as possible over their lifespan, there is a need to reduce and eliminate systematic differences in the health of groups and communities. The application of the highest-quality research from a lifespan developmental approach in studying outcomes related to health and disease combined with the empirical study and systematic policy analyses of the regulations and laws that affect health equity are essential to reduce health disparities and improve health equity and justice.

THE CHARACTER ASSASSINATION OF BLACK MALES: SOME CONSEQUENCES FOR RESEARCH IN PUBLIC HEALTH

Authors: Alford A. Young, Jr., PhD

A consequence of pervasive social inequality is the regard by those of higher socioeconomic standing of those at the bottom of American social hierarchies, especially men and boys of color, as unworthy citizens. Many people believe that the poor have brought their condition upon themselves as a consequence of being embedded in moral, cultural, and biological deficiencies. African American males register in the minds of the American public as threatening, hostile, aggressive, unconscientious, and incorrigible. Beliefs about their moral and cultural short-comings help engineer a warped vision not only of their capacities for positive individual and collective action, but of their very public identities.

Bearing the mark of unworthiness and the accompanying social undesirability that comes from it subjects African American males to an extreme form of character assassination. A character assassination is an act of consistently presenting false or indicting arguments about a person in order to encourage his or her public dislike or mistrust.

For example, black males do not necessarily reject mainstream institutional spheres such as schools but rather have negative experiences with individuals in these spheres. The result is that they face problems with their encounters with schools, employers, and legal authorities such as the police, but not with schooling, employment, or the institution of law in a general sense.

Media coverage of public debates following the deaths of numerous African American males in recent years has centered on two forms of public response and inquiry. One was whether these individuals conducted themselves as proper or deserving people. The other was whether they appeared to be highly threatening or dangerous in the moments prior to their deaths. Implicit in these and other tragic deaths of such males was the notion that what they did, who they were, or how they appeared to be at the time in which they were approached by those who encountered them was credible explanation, if not complete justification, for what transpired.

The health consequences of racism include various forms of trauma which affect the psychological and physiological states of being in these males. The existence of character assassination may not result in any explicit impingement upon individual behavior or conduct. However, the extreme surveillance of and critical social judgement made about the conduct, action, or dispositions exemplified by black males may be causal factors for a range of unhealthy emotional and physical states of being. Ultimately, any wholesale mitigation of the character assassination of these males can only occur if there is a shift in the public imagination of them.

PROMOTING POSITIVE DEVELOPMENT, HEALTH, AND SOCIAL JUSTICE THROUGH DISMANTLING GENETIC DETERMINISM

AUTHORS: RICHARD M. LERNER, PhD

Reductionist, genetic determinist ideas have created inequities in access to individual social resources and opportunities. As a result, these ideas have created inequities in health, education, and social justice. Social justice focuses on social inequities, characterized as avoidable and unjust social structures and policies that limit access to resources based solely on group or individual characteristics such as race/ethnicity, age, gender, sexual orientation, physical or developmental ability status, and/or immigration status, among others. Social justice emphasizes the rights of all groups in society to have fair access to and a voice in policies governing the distribution of resources essential to their physical and psychological well-being.

Modern genetic determinist ideas suggest that genes account for racial differences in wealth and economic institutions and disregard the effects of the social determinants of health (i.e., discrimination, racism, and lack of education). However, human development has the capacity for plasticity, which contradicts the notion that genes preclude individuals from profiting from health or education programs. An alternative to genetic determinism is the relational developmental systems (RDS) metamodel which embraces a new understanding of the role of biology in human development. The RDS metamodel is predicated on an integrative understanding of evolution and epigenetics. The conceptual emphasis in these theories is placed on a mutually influential relationship between individuals and their contexts. Thus biological, psychological, and behavioral attributes of the person, combined with culture, have a temporal (historical) component. For example, the genome of infants can be modified by epigenetic changes involving experiential and environmental variables, and this modification can be transmitted across generations.

Developmental science can be used to accurately reflect the diversity of human development; dismantle modern notions of genetic determinism; and build bridges across various disciplines, professions, and communities to ensure integrative, multidisciplinary, collaborative approaches to promoting human health and social justice.

PHILOSOPHICAL PERSPECTIVES ON SOCIAL JUSTICE: A FRAMEWORK FOR DISCUSSING A CHILDREN, YOUTH, AND FAMILIES HEALTH POLICY AND RESEARCH AGENDA

AUTHORS: ROBERT SEIDEL, MLA, PATRICK H. TOLAN, PhD, ANGELA DIAZ, MD, PhD, MPH, AND VELMA McBRIDE MURRY, PhD

Discussions on social justice and health equity often assume that stakeholders have universally agreed upon definitions of these two concepts and adhere to a certain set of foundational principles. However, outside of academic circles, the ideas of "social justice" and "health equity" are rarely articulated, and people may have differing views of what these ideas mean and their role in furthering health policy agendas. In the American context, greater clarification of these terms can acknowledge implicit variations in our values and assumptions and better benefit efforts to achieve effective health policy. Various philosophical schools of thought have many definitions of social justice and ideals for how people should interact and how communities should allocate resources. In discussing social justice and health equity, the two major categories of philosophical perspectives are "individual-centric," which emphasize the rights and well-being of the individual, and "community-centric," which emphasize the well-being of the community or society.

"Individual-centric" perspectives share similarities with the prevailing American political philosophy of liberalism, a central concern for the protection and enhancement of the freedom of individuals. More specifically, traditional American liberalism seeks to realize the promises of the U.S. Constitution to all people regardless of natural or social differences; this philosophy has been demonstrated in movements to attain civil rights for women, African Americans, and LGBTQ+ people. Libertarianism favors an abundance of choice, personal agency, and a reduction in government regulation over initiatives for equal opportunity, but this perspective also argues that increasing individual choice will lead to greater justice. Rawls' concept of justice as fairness believes that policies and resources should be targeted toward the reduction of inequities in society. Nussbaum and Sen's capabilities approach moves past typical conceptions of human rights and posits that differential opportunity is necessary to compensate for inherent disadvantages among people.

"Community-centric" perspectives are associated with the majority of cultures in human history and give primacy to the success of an overall society over the individual. Tribal social organization principles require contributions from all to a society's productivity, while ensuring the equal status of every individual in the community. Confucianism proposes that the moral conduct of individuals engenders political order, and that personal identity is defined by a person's relationships. Buddhism understands the interdependency of people and warns that ignoring the plight of the poor leads to negative effects for all of society. Utilitarianism, based on the idea of maximizing benefits, is problematic in discussing health equity due to differing judgments of the meaning of "good" and the means by which this good can be achieved. Socialism and communism can be seen to some extent in nationalized health insurance systems in Europe and deserve further consideration from the American perspective.

By investigating various philosophical perspectives on social justice more deeply, Americans can prioritize their values regarding individual liberties, government regulation, community interdependency, and resource allocation. This understanding of our values would, in turn, strengthen our debates over the role of social justice and health equity in our society and support the creation of better policies and programs in health care.

EXPULSION AND SUSPENSION IN EARLY EDUCATION AS MATTERS OF SOCIAL JUSTICE AND HEALTH EQUITY

AUTHORS: SHANTEL E. MEEK, PhD, AND WALTER S. GILLIAM, PhD

Social justice—equal access and opportunity for all—has been a core American value since our founding. That value, however, is not fully realized in the lives of millions of Americans, nor has it ever been. Scientists have a central role in addressing the challenges that face society. A primary purpose of research should be to inform the policies and practices that in turn address serious problems in our country and around the world. Racial, ethnic, socioeconomic, and ability-based disparities and inequities are widespread across most aspects of society. These disparities start early, perhaps before birth, and are pervasive throughout children's lives before they even enter kindergarten.

It is well established that the beginning years of any child's life are critical for building the early foundation needed for success in school and later in life. During this period, the brain develops at a pace unlike any other, and is extraordinarily sensitive to and affected by children's environments, experiences, and relationships. Early adversities can have lasting consequences—and these adversities (and the protective buffers) are inequitably distributed.

Low-income children and children of color alike have less access to high-quality early learning programs. Young boys of color are especially more likely to be pushed out of early childhood programs through exclusionary practices like suspension and expulsion. While African American children make up 18 percent of preschool enrollment, they make up 48 percent of preschoolers suspended. Early expulsion and suspension predict later expulsion and suspension, and students who are expelled or suspended are as much as 10 times more likely to drop out of high school, experience academic failure and grade retention, hold negative school attitudes, and face incarceration than those who are not. Expulsion and suspension are pivotal points of influence in young children's lives that may contribute to entry into the "prison pipeline" and therefore must be immediately addressed by a broad coalition of stakeholders, including researchers; policy makers; and local districts, schools, and community-based programs.

Understanding the degree to which implicit biases may contribute to expulsion and suspension decisions by early educators and administrators is an important step to a fuller understanding of the source of disciplinary disparities. No intervention to date has targeted, examined, and published findings on reducing or eliminating the racial disparities noted in expulsion and suspension data in early childhood settings, which is a clear and pressing need.

LESSONS FOR HEALTH EQUITY: MILITARY MEDICINE AS A WINDOW TO UNIVERSAL HEALTH INSURANCE

Authors: Jeff Hutchinson, MD, FAAP, Raquel Mack, MS, Tracey Pérez Koehlmoos, PhD, MHA, and Patrick H. DeLeon, PhD, MPH, JD

Health disparities result from multifaceted variables including access to health care, and discrimination associated with socioeconomic status, education, social support, insurance, race, ethnicity, and gender. The purpose of this paper is to identify lessons learned and future research opportunities from the two national health systems that model universal health care, the Military Health System (MHS), and the Department of Veterans Affairs (VA).

The federal health care system provides an excellent vehicle for objectively exploring the underlying determinants of health disparities. The Military Health System primarily serves the active duty population, their family members as well as some retirees, whereas the VA exclusively treats veterans—a generally older cohort. The differences in health outcomes are influenced by the different patient populations, organization structure, and priority. The similarities in disparities that have decreased are most likely the result of electronic medical record use, similar provider cohorts, and a single insurer. Increased focus on these health care delivery systems has the potential to clarify sources and solutions to health disparities.

The data available from the VA and MHS demonstrate both elimination of disparities and areas where disparities continue despite equal access and resources. Cultural factors of disparities arise from gender, religion, race, ethnicity, and any shared group experience. Theoretically, the traditional barriers of access, patient and provider economic concerns, and provider shortages should explain disparate outcomes. Race-based, cultural distrust of military medicine is not eliminated immediately upon entering the service. Ongoing research indicates a lack of disparities across a variety of health and surgical-related access and outcomes including maternal, cancer, and heart surgical procedures. However, several biases remain in place even after universal coverage eliminates access and resource discrepancies. Other areas that continue to demonstrate disparities require exploration of new variables that contribute to health disparities (such as rank and service) to improve military and veteran health care.

PRINCIPLES OF ADOLESCENT- AND YOUNG-ADULT-FRIENDLY CARE: CONTRIBUTIONS TO REDUCING HEALTH DISPARITIES AND INCREASING HEALTH EQUITY

AUTHORS: ANGELA DIAZ, MD, PhD, MPH, AND KEN PEAKE, DSW

The behavioral patterns that evolve during adolescence help determine young people's immediate health status and influence their long-term health, including their risk for developing chronic diseases in adulthood, and which can result in health disparities further down the road. During adolescence, the responsibility to be healthy begins to shift from caregivers to young people, making it critical to ensure that young people have access to health care, education, and the opportunity to develop the skills they need to be productive and make valuable societal contributions. Many young people lack health literacy and have no experience navigating the silos by which health care is organized. Health care providers can play a unique role in providing appropriate interventions that encourage young people to become great health care consumers and adopt healthy behaviors.

Despite the opportunity that adolescence presents for health care systems to shape future well-being, the current health care delivery system is not sufficient in addressing the needs of young people. Historically adolescents have long received less health care than other age groups, even after the implementation of the Affordable Care Act. A key challenge that will shape adolescent health in the next decade is presented by the fact that the adolescent population is becoming more ethnically diverse. The growing diversity of young people involved in the health care system will demand cultural responsiveness if health care needs are to be properly met.

In recognition of the unique developmental characteristics, concerns, opportunities for health promotion and vulnerabilities of adolescents, along with their relative inexperience in seeking or navigating health care independently, there is an emerging consensus about the principles that should guide the design and delivery of adolescent health services. These principles include equitable care; reaching out to those most vulnerable; accessible and easily navigated care; integrated services; confidential care; informed consent; developmentally appropriate care; relationship-based care; supporting one-on-one youth provider interactions; sensitive, trained, and reflective staff; creating a safe space that is nonjudgmental; respectful care; culturally competent care; and promoting parent-child communication. These principles can be used in adolescent- and young-adult-specific health centers to understand and mitigate disparities related to lack of access, poor quality of services, or services that are inadequate.

STORIES ABOUT BLACK MEN IN THE MEDIA AND THEIR CONSEQUENCES FOR HEALTH

AUTHORS: KAREN E. DILL-SHACKLEFORD, PHD, SRIVIDYA RAMASUBRAMANIAN, PHD, MA, AND LAWRENCE M. DRAKE II, PHD, MA, MPA

At this particular juncture in U.S. history, the fictional entertainment and news media stories we tell about black men are vitally important to our individual and collective development as a society. Despite the progress of black males in education, industry, and other areas of America's landscape, the media continues to highlight a negative narrative that associates black men with violence, crime, and poverty. In the media, black men are overrepresented as street criminals and underrepresented in positive social roles and in positions of power. A number of studies have demonstrated that the stories we tell about black men in the media have negative consequences such as increased prejudice and decreased support for pro-black ideas and policies.

News reports often use subtle cues and visual codes that rationalize white superiority and present black men as disruptive and troublesome. Research documents that news stories about black men often attribute their failures to personal deficiencies such as incompetence or lack of motivation, rather than to systemic factors such as discrimination or lack of access to quality education, employment, and health care. Simply bringing to mind a stereotype or counter-stereotype is sufficient to influence subsequent judgments, beliefs, and behavioral intentions.

Apart from encouraging diverse and positive portrayals of black men in mainstream media, it is important to foster alternative media spaces for black voices to be amplified and heard. The Black Lives Matter (BLM) movement began after a series of events involving mistreatment, mishandling, or violence toward African Americans by white police officers and their authorities. The BLM movement offers a perspective on how to plot the use of technology-based communication platforms to expose the injustice of the violence being perpetrated while unifying their message.

A growing number of researchers have argued that pervasive racism, including race-laced messages fostered by the media, has an adverse impact on the health conditions of blacks and other racial minorities. The stigmatization of black men extends to the health domain because prejudice and discrimination have been shown to elevate depression and anxiety, with cascading effects on numerous chronic illnesses. The factors are often characterized as social determinants of health and contribute to racial health disparities. When we tell false stories about an entire demographic, we cause stress and ill health and even aggression in not only that demographic, but in others who encounter them.

It is important to become aware of the detrimental ways media stories shape our idea about the world and ourselves. Efforts to intervene can occur through media literacy education to educate the public to become informed media consumers. Most research studies on media effects generally focus on majority participants and the segments of our population who enjoy more privilege. Therefore, more research is needed that gives voice to minority participants. It is imperative that we find space in our schools to educate our children in media literacy. This would allow for dialogue about responsibility for messaging and for responding to messaging that is derogatory to any one race.

History has made it abundantly clear that shared cultural stereotypes of black men are contributing to brutality and injustice towards black men. Popular media have been part of the problem in perpetuating negative race-related messages, forestalling resolutions to racial tensions in our society. As we look for opportunities for positive change, there is evidence to suggest that including popular media in the solution is a viable option.

CHALLENGES AND PROMISE OF HEALTH EQUITY FOR NATIVE HAWAIIANS

Authors: Noreen Mokuau, DSW, Patrick H. DeLeon, PhD, MPH, JD, Joseph Keawe'aimoku Kaholokula, PhD, Sadé Soares, JoAnn U. Tsark, MPH, and Coti-Lynne Puamana Haia, JD

Health equity, the attainment of the highest level of health for all people, is yet to be realized for many populations in the United States. Health equity focuses on diseases and health care services, but is also broadly linked to social determinants, such as socioeconomic status, the physical environment, discrimination, and legislative policies. For Native Hawaiians, the indigenous people of Hawai'i, the elusiveness of health equity is reflected in the excess burden of health and social disparities.

Native Hawaiians make up approximately 21 percent of the state's multiethnic population of 1.4 million. The cumulative impact of the colonization, oppression, and cultural suppression of Native Hawaiians during the 19th and 20th centuries has subjugated them to long-term injustice and discrimination. The historical loss of population, land, culture, and self-identity has shaped the economic and psychosocial landscape of Hawai'i's people, and limits their ability to actualize optimal health.

Consequently, Native Hawaiians have the shortest life expectancy and exhibit higher mortality rates than the total population due to heart disease, cancer, stroke, and diabetes. Poor health is inextricably linked to socioeconomic factors, and Native Hawaiians are more likely to live below the poverty level, experience higher rates of unemployment, live in crowded and impoverished conditions, and experience imprisonment.

Native Hawaiians' cultural values and beliefs are organized around the collective relationships of the family, community, land, and spiritual realm. Therefore, effective interventions will incorporate these beliefs. There are various model programs that have the potential to impact health through policies that increase the Native Hawaiian workforce in health care; tailor research to specifically examine and treat health disparities among Native Hawaiians; and develop new clinical interventions that are community-based and culturally anchored.

For Native Hawaiians to eventually achieve health equity there must be (1) an institutional commitment by universities to train a sufficient number of Native Hawaiians in all disciplines to address health disparities and create health solutions; (2) the establishment of culturally sensitive health care systems which will affirmatively seek out Native Hawaiian patients; and (3) a serious appreciation for the complexity of Native Hawaiian culture at the policy level.

FETAL ALCOHOL SPECTRUM DISORDERS IN AFRICAN AMERICAN COMMUNITIES: CONTINUING THE QUEST FOR PREVENTION

Author: Carl C. Bell, MD

Over the past decade, public health research has placed an increasing emphasis on prevention. However, a major piece of the dialogue has been overlooked: fetal alcohol exposure (FAE). Several diagnoses fall under the category of fetal alcohol spectrum disorders (FASD)—the overarching diagnosis that is caused by FAE. Thanks to public health efforts by the Centers for Disease Control and Prevention, National Institute on Alcohol Abuse and Alcoholism, and Substance Abuse and Mental Health Services Administration, the knowledge that women should not drink during pregnancy is nearly ubiquitous. Unfortunately, a large proportion of women are drinking socially before they realize they are pregnant. This is further supported by the fact that nearly 50 percent of pregnancies are unplanned. Additionally, women 18–24 years old, who are poor, have unintended pregnancy rates 2–3 times higher than the national average. The consequence of alcohol consumption during pregnancy is birthing a child with fetal alcohol spectrum. There is a higher likelihood of FASD cases in African American communities, partly due to the increased access to alcohol because of the overabundance of liquor stores in the African American community.

Numerous disorders have been associate with FASD, exhibited in varying degrees of impaired growth, including cognitive and behavioral abnormalities and facial abnormalities. Future problems may include learning disabilities; school performance deficits; inadequate impulse control; social perceptual problems; language dysfunction; abstraction difficulties; mathematics deficiencies; and judgment, memory, and attention problems.

FASD produces an acquired biological disability of subtle brain damage. This subtle brain damage masquerades as a whole host of educational, criminal, and psychiatric disorders. These children's adversities are further exacerbated, as many of them are also victimized and/or exposed to violence at a young age. The combination of biological and environmental risk is often viewed as the central factor that places youth at risk for numerous disparities. For example, given the likelihood of dysregulatory behaviors among FASD children, it is highly probable that their behavior may be misdiagnosed, setting them up for early entry into the juvenile justice system. Although the intellectual and behavioral symptoms of FASD have been attributed to culture in African Americans, the reality is that these behaviors are caused by the social determinants of health that put them at risk for subtle brain damage.

While medical students, historically, have been taught to look for fetal alcohol facies in infants, that the problem has long-term effects over a child's life course suggests the need to shift to a paradigm. For example, the American Psychiatric Association has included a diagnosis of neurobehavioral disorder associated with prenatal alcohol exposure (ND-PAE) in DSM-5. It is possible that the most common problems occurring in all youth—1) speech and language disorders, 2) specific learning disorders, 3) ADHD, and 4) mild intellectual deficiency originated with FASD. FASD awareness is hampered by the lack of understanding that efforts can be undertaken to intervene. Results from animal studies have demonstrated that a choline supplement during pregnancy and postnatally can reduce the damage done to fetuses that have been exposed to alcohol, but human clinical trials have been lagging behind. Despite all the progress in public health, there is an urgent need to bring to the forefront the consequences for children born to mothers who use alcohol during pregnancy.

URGENT DISPATCH: CALLING ON LEADERSHIP TO RESPOND TO VIOLENCE IN BLACK NEIGHBORHOODS AS A PUBLIC HEALTH CRISIS

Authors: Sharon Toomer and Raquel Mack, MS

People in black neighborhoods across the nation are plagued with unceasing and prolonged violence. There is a failure to target and respond to this public health crisis and social and health injustice. Numerous women, men, girls, and boys are left to navigate the long-term psychosocial effects of continued violence. Violence in black neighborhoods is a public health crisis that requires immediate, decisive, targeted, and swift action involving all sectors in a position to respond with expertise, leadership, and resources.

Community violence is defined as exposure to intentional acts of interpersonal violence committed in public areas by individuals who are not intimately related to the victim. Living under a stagnant cloud of community violence is traumatizing and the immediate and long-term impact of community violence is recognizable. Community violence has a strong impact on the mental health outcomes of children and adolescents. Exposure to violent death causes psychological trauma and can result in complicated grief disorder, which involves extreme immobilization, pronounced psychotic ideation and severe symptoms that persist over a long passage of time. This can also cause a breakdown in psychological functioning. Being in a state of shock, experiencing denial, avoidance or loss reminders, and dysfunctional or health-compromising behaviors are indicators of complicated grief. Consequently, black people are at a greater risk of developing complicated grief disorder because they experience homicide more frequently than the majority population and have elevated grief symptoms in comparison. The effects of trauma are also generational, which supports the case that an immediate and targeted public health response to violence is essential to the well-being and progress of those affected.

Undeniably the United States is a violent nation and violence does not discriminate based on socioeconomic status, race, or ethnicity. But the especially chilling rate and frequency of violence happening in black neighborhoods, and the unaddressed trauma that follow, is discriminate. Until there is the political and societal will to comprehensively analyze, examine, address, and, more urgently, remedy the factors leading to the present-day conditions, violence will continue to plague black neighborhoods across the nation.

So far, law enforcement, the criminal justice system and more punitive measures through legislation (e.g., gun laws) have been the driving solution. But those systems and measures have not curbed the violence and they do not address the emotional and mental health needs of traumatized people in black neighborhoods. The essential and immediate need is a declared public health crisis followed by targeted, multifaceted action and resources.

APPENDIX B

The Board on Children, Youth, and Families
Spring Board Meeting Agenda

National Academy of Sciences, Keck Center
500 Fifth Street, NW, Keck 100
Washington, DC 20001
Monday, May 11, 2015

ARMCHAIR DISCUSSIONS OF SOCIAL JUSTICE AND EQUITY ACROSS THE LIFE COURSE

Meeting Objectives:

1. Address current laws, policies, and the leadership needed to ensure social justice and equity for children, youth, and families.
2. Highlight "institutions" such as parenting, the juvenile justice system, foster care system, school system, and ways these institutions protect the development of children and youth in the context of social justice and equity.
3. Focus on disparities resulting from discriminatory practices and policies, and missed opportunities for not investing in human capital.
4. Discuss topics and priority areas for the IOM.

12:30 PM   Slam poetry videos highlighting multiple perspectives

12:35 pm   Welcome Remarks

Velma McBride Murry, Meeting Chair, Vanderbilt University

12:40 PM   Opening comments from Victor Dzau, President of the Institute of Medicine

12:50 PM   Panel 1—The legal landscape for social justice and equity

Objective: Speakers in this session will address current laws, policies, and the leadership needed to ensure social justice and equity for children, youth, and families.

Chair/Moderator: Pat DeLeon, Uniformed Services University of the Health Services

Speakers:
- Bruce Lesley, First Focus
- Eugene Steuerle, The Urban Institute
- Carl Bell, University of Illinois at Chicago
- Terry Flood, Jubilee Jobs
- Spero Manson, University of Colorado at Denver
- Bill Whitner, Miriam's Kitchen

Research Reaction: Patrick Tolan, Youth-Nex, University of Virginia

1:45 PM   Panel 2—Institutions through the life course

Objective: This session will highlight "institutions" such as parenting, the juvenile-justice system, foster-care system, school system, and ways these institutions protect the development of children and youth in the context of social justice and equity.

Chair/Moderator: Vivian Gadsden, National Center on Fathers and Families, University of Pennsylvania

Speakers:
- Oscar Barbarin, Tulane University
- Maria Cancian, U.S. Department of Health and Human Services
- Harry Holzer, Brookings Institution
- Irasema Salcido, Founder, Cesar Chavez Charter Schools for Public Policy (Washington, DC)
- Adriana Umana-Taylor, Arizona State University
- Mark Courtney, University of Chicago
- Jeff Hutchinson, Uniformed Services University of the Health Sciences
- Ruth Lubic, Developing Families Center, Inc. and Family Health Birth Center

Research Reaction: Dara Blachman-Demner, National Institute of Justice

3:00 PM **BREAK**

3:15 PM **Panel 3—Consequences of inequality on loss of human capital**

Objective: Discussions will focus on disparities resulting from discriminatory practices and policies, and missed opportunities for not investing in human capital.

Chair/Moderator: Margaret Beale Spencer, University of Chicago

Speakers:
- Hernan Carvente, Vera Institute
- Larke Huang, Substance Abuse and Mental Health Services Administration
- Richard Lerner, Tufts University
- Nancy Lopez, University of New Mexico
- Martin Sepulveda, IBM
- Alford Young Jr., University of Michigan

Research Reactions:
Eve Reider, National Center for Complementary & Integrative Health
Belinda Sims, National Institute on Drug Abuse

4:15 PM **BREAKOUT SESSION**

Objective: Table groups will discuss future topics and priority areas for the IOM. Tables will be arranged to include individuals from varying sectors.

5:00 PM **Report Out**

5:45 PM **Closing Remarks**

Velma McBride Murry, Meeting Chair, Vanderbilt University
Angela Diaz, BCYF Board Chair, Mount Sinai School of Medicine

6:00 PM **Adjourn**

APPENDIX C

Program of "Engaging Allies in the Culture of Health Movement"

National Academy of Medicine

Stakeholder Meeting #1
January 25, 2017
Keck Center, Room 100
500 Fifth Street NW
Washington, DC 20001

Note Regarding Today's Meeting

The purpose of today's meeting is to share information about strategies for achieving health equity rather than the discussion of specific legislation at the state or federal level that may be relevant to this topic. Because this gathering is funded by the Robert Wood Johnson Foundation and there are government representatives in the room, we ask that you avoid references to specific federal or state pending or proposed legislation.

Wednesday January 25, 2017   Open Session   Keck 100

8:00 AM   Networking Breakfast

8:30 AM   Welcome

Kimber Bogard, Managing Officer, Culture of Health Program, National Academy of Medicine

8:45 AM   Live Performance

Adam Booth, Words Artist and Musician, Appalachia

243

9:00 AM   Opening Remarks

Victor Dzau, President National Academy of Medicine

9:15 AM   Poll Everywhere

Charlee Alexander, Associate Program Officer, National Academy of Medicine
Q: What is the most important health equity issue to you or your organization?

9:30 AM   Views from the Robert Wood Johnson Foundation

James Marks, Executive VP, RWJF

9:45 AM   Health equity crosses boundaries

Discussion Moderator: Raynard Kington, President, Grinnell College
- **William Valiant & Emad Madha**, Uniformed Services University of the Health Sciences
- **Alexander Billioux**, Acting Director, Division of Population Health Incentives and Infrastructure, Preventive & Population Health Group, Center for Medicare & Medicaid Innovation

10:20 AM   Keynote

What is the current state of the science on early-life inequities and its limitations in informing how to achieve health equity for all?

Discussion Moderator: Stuart Butler, Brookings Institution
- **Sarah Watamura**, Associate Professor, Department of Psychology, University of Denver
- **Valerie Maholmes**, Chief of the Pediatric Trauma and Critical Illness Branch, National Institute of Child Health and Human Development

11:00 AM   Break & Poll Everywhere for input and comments on keynote talk

Ivory Clarke, Research Assistant, National Academies of Sciences, Engineering, and Medicine
Q: What social determinants of health stand out to you in your work or community?

11:15 AM   Health Equity report findings and recommendations

- **Rose Martinez**, Senior Director, Board on Population Health, Health and Medicine Division
- **Alison Evans Cuellar**, Professor, Health Administration & Policy, George Mason University
- **Helene Gayle**, CEO, McKinsey Social Initiative

11:45 AM   What is the role of community data in achieving optimal health for all?

Thomas Mason, Chief Medical Officer, Office of the National Coordinator for Health Information Technology

12:00 PM   Lunchtime discussion

Q: What opportunities do you have to build health equity in your community, state, research? Who are the community members that may be overlooked?

12:45 PM   Panel

Q: How can we accelerate progress in health equity across settings and sectors?

Discussion Moderator: Antonia Villarruel, Margaret Bond Simon Dean of Nursing, University of Pennsylvania

1. A. Military
Col. Jeff Hutchinson, Associate Dean, Clinical Affairs/Chief Diversity Officer, Uniformed Services University of the Health Sciences

1. B. Business & Industry
Robert Dugger, Board Member, Council for a Strong America; CoFounder and Advisory Board Chair, ReadyNation; Founder & Managing Partner, Hanover Investment, L.L.C.

2. A. State government
John Dreyzehner, Commissioner, TN Department of Health

2. B. Community
Gretchen Musicant, Minneapolis Health Commissioner

3. A. Philanthropy
Tara Westman, Program Manager, Southern California Region, The California Endowment

3. B. Research
Vivian Gadsden, Director, National Center on Fathers and Families and Professor of Child Development and Education, University of Pennsylvania Graduate School of Education

2:00 PM   Discussion

Moderator: **Dwayne Proctor,** Director and Senior Adviser, Robert Wood Johnson Foundation

2:30 PM   Standing break/Poll Everywhere

Ivory Clarke, Research Assistant, National Academies of Sciences, Engineering, and Medicine
   Q: *What do you still need to know to accelerate progress in health equity in your community/state/at the federal level?*

2:45 PM   Call to action

Helene Gayle, *CEO, McKinsey Social Initiative*

3:00 PM   Adjourn open session

NAM CULTURE OF HEALTH PROGRAM
ADVISORY GROUP

- Hortensia de los Angeles Amaro, PhD
- Stuart Butler, PhD
- Angela Diaz, MD
- John Dreyzehner, MD
- Shirley Franklin
- Julian Harris, MD, MBA
- Jeff Hutchinson, MD
- Otho Kerr, JD
- Raynard Kington, MD, PhD
- Howard K. Koh, MD, MPH
- Velma McBride Murry, PhD
- Dwayne Proctor, PhD
- Karen Remley, MD, MBA, MPH, FAAP
- Anna Ricklin, MHS
- Martin Sepulveda, MD, ScD
- Tipiziwin Tolman
- Antonia M. Villarruel, PhD, RN, FAAN

APPENDIX D

AUTHOR BIOGRAPHIES

Carl C. Bell, MD, is Staff Psychiatrist at Jackson Park Hospital's Outpatient Family Practice Clinic and Inpatient Consultation Liaison Service. He is the Chairman of the Department of Psychiatry, Windsor University, St. Kitts. In addition, he is a Professor Emeritus, Psychiatry, Department of Psychiatry, School of Medicine and Retired Clinical Professor of Psychiatry & Public Health at the University of Illinois at Chicago. During 50 years, he has published more than 575 articles, chapters, and books on mental health and authored The Sanity of Survival. He is coeditor of *Family and HIV/AIDS: Cultural and Contextual Issues in Prevention and Treatment* and *Psychiatric Clinics of North America—Prevention in Psychiatry*. He is a member of the Executive Committee of the National Action Alliance for the Prevention of Suicide. In 2012, he was presented the Special Presidential Commendation of the American Psychiatric Association in recognition of his outstanding advocacy for mental illness prevention and for person-centered mental health wellness and recovery, and the 2012 Agnes Purcell McGavin Award for Prevention in Child and Adolescent Psychiatry. In 2014, he was presented the American Psychiatric Association's Distinguished Service Award and the Abraham Halpern Humanitarian Award from the American Association of Social Psychiatry.

Patrick H. DeLeon, PhD, MPH, JD, is a Distinguished Professor at the Uniformed Services University of the Health Sciences Daniel K. Inouye Graduate School of Nursing (GSN) and the F. Edward Hebert School of Medicine. As a Distinguished Professor for the Daniel K. Inouye Graduate School of Nursing, Dr. DeLeon leads the Public Policy Forum, where numerous distinguished visitors and delegates are invited to speak. A few of his career highlights include working for the Peace Corps, and as a Public Health intern for Senator Daniel K. Inouye. Remarkably, Dr. DeLeon's internship turned into a 38-year term of public service in support of strengthening access to care and health policies for the Hawaiian culture, and retiring as Chief of Staff to Senator Inouye in 2011.

Preeminently, Dr. DeLeon was instrumental in standing up the GSN, and he is considered one of its founding fathers. Dr. DeLeon has been awarded three honorary degrees: honorary doctor of psychology from the California School of Professional Psychology, Fresno; honorary doctor of psychology from the Forest Institute of Professional Psychology; and an honorary doctor of humane letters from NOVA Southeastern University. He is currently the editor of *Psychological Services*. He has over 200 publications. He is married with one son, a daughter, one grandson, and one granddaughter. In his spare time, he enjoys writing and playing golf.

Angela Diaz, MD, PhD, MPH, is the Jean C. and James W. Crystal Professor in Adolescent Health and Professor of Pediatrics and Preventive Medicine at the Icahn School of Medicine. After earning her medical degree at Columbia University College of Physicians and Surgeons, she completed her postdoctoral training at the Mount Sinai School of Medicine and subsequently received a master's in public health from Harvard University and PhD in epidemiology from Columbia University. Dr. Diaz is the Director of the Mount Sinai Adolescent Health Center, a unique program that provides high quality, comprehensive, integrated, interdisciplinary primary care, sexual and reproductive health, mental health, dental and health education services to teens—all for free to those without insurance. The Center has an emphasis on wellness and prevention. Under her leadership, the Center has become the largest, adolescent-specific health center in the United States, serving each year more than 10,000 vulnerable and disadvantaged youth, including those who are uninsured and lack access to health services. This program addresses health disparity and aims for health equity.

Karen Dill-Shackleford, PhD, earned her PhD in social psychology from the University of Missouri-Columbia. Her dissertation on media violence has been cited 1,500 times. She testified twice before Congress about media use and everyday realities. Karen studies the way people seek and construct social meaning from media including fictional stories, especially in the context of fandom. She demonstrates how media can be used to enhance social justice, particularly related to issues involving race and gender. She also studies the benefits of using media to support a meditation practice to enhance psychological well-being. Karen is the author of *How Fantasy Becomes Reality*, and the editor of the *Oxford Handbook of Media Psychology*. She is coauthor of *Mad Men Unzipped: Fans on Sex, Love, and the Sixties on TV* (University of Iowa Press, 2015); and *Finding Truth in Fiction: The Benefits of Getting Lost in a Story* (Oxford University Press, 2015).

Lawrence M. Drake II, PhD, MA, MPA, currently serves and President and Chief Executive Officer of the Leadership, Education, and Development (LEAD) Program and is responsible for the overall operational and strategic leadership of the organization. Dr. Drake serves as chairman of Hope 360°, an executive management advisory firm. He is a certified consultant for Personnel Decisions International, an investment adviser for AJIA Capital Holdings, and is a senior partner at Saurus Partners LLC. He retired from The Coca-Cola Company where he was managing director, President/CEO of the $1B West Africa division of Coca-Cola Africa. Previously, he served in senior-level positions with Executive Leadership Council, PepsiCo, Cablevision Systems Corp., and Kraft Inc. He has helped bring several start-ups/midstage entrepreneurial companies to market, including Haven Media Group and Dolman Technologies. He serves or has served on the boards and executive committees of the National Conference for Community and Justice, the California Science Center, Crystal Stairs Inc., Jarvis Christian College, the Executive Leadership Council, Vine & Oak Foundation North America, and Nehemiah Project Ministries International. He received a BA in sociology from Georgia State University and an MBA from Rockhurst University, where he was an executive fellow. Mr. Drake completed both his MA and PhD in psychology at Fielding Graduate University in Santa Barbara, California.

Vivian L. Gadsden, EdD, is the William T. Carter Professor of Child Development, Professor of Education, and Director of the National Center on Fathers and Families at the University of Pennsylvania. She is also on the faculties of Africana Studies and of Gender, Sexuality, and Women's Studies at Penn. Gadsden is President of the American Educational Research Association. Gadsden's research and scholarly interests focus on children and families across the life course who are at the greatest risk for academic and social vulnerability by virtue of race, gender, ethnicity, poverty, and immigrant status. Her current projects examine young children's learning and well-being; parenting and family engagement, including father involvement; health and educational disparities within low-income communities; and incarceration and its effects on children and families. She serves on the Board of the Foundation for Child Development and on a range of national and local research initiatives. Most recently, she served as chair of The National Academies of Sciences, Engineering, and Medicine's Committee on Supporting Parents of Young Children. Gadsden is a Fellow of the American Educational Research Association. She earned her doctorate in education and developmental psychology from the University of Michigan.

Helene D. Gayle is president and CEO of The Chicago Community Trust. Before assuming leadership of the Trust in October 2017, Dr. Gayle was CEO of McKinsey Social Initiative, a nonprofit that brings together varied stakeholders to address complex global social challenges. From 2006 to 2015, she was president and CEO of CARE USA, a leading international humanitarian organization. An expert on global development, humanitarian and health issues, Dr. Gayle spent 20 years with the Centers for Disease Control and Prevention, working primarily on HIV/AIDS. She also worked at the Bill & Melinda Gates Foundation, directing programs on HIV/AIDS and other global health issues. Dr. Gayle serves on public company and nonprofit boards including the Coca-Cola Company, Colgate-Palmolive Company, the Rockefeller Foundation, Brookings Institution, the Center for Strategic and International Studies, New America, and the ONE Campaign. She is a member of the Council on Foreign Relations, the American Public Health Association, the National Academy of Medicine, the National Medical Association and the American Academy of Pediatrics. Named one of *Forbes'* "100 Most Powerful Women," she has authored numerous articles on global and domestic public health issues, poverty alleviation, gender equality and social justice. Dr. Gayle was born and raised in Buffalo, New York. She earned a BA in psychology at Barnard College, an M.D. at the University of Pennsylvania and an MPH at Johns Hopkins University. She has received 13 honorary degrees and holds faculty appointments at the University of Washington and Emory University.

Walter S. Gilliam, PhD, is the Director of The Edward Zigler Center in Child Development and Social Policy and associate professor of child psychiatry and psychology at the Child Study Center, Yale School of Medicine. He is on the board of directors for the National Association of Child Care Resource and Referral Agencies (NACCRRA), a fellow at Zero to Three and the National Institute for Early Education Research (NIEER), and served as a senior advisor to the National Association for the Education of Young Children (NAEYC). Dr. Gilliam is corecipient of the 2008 Grawemeyer Award in Education for the coauthored book, *A Vision for Universal Preschool Education*. Dr. Gilliam's research involves early childhood education and intervention policy analysis (specifically how policies translate into effective services), ways to improve the quality of prekindergarten and childcare services, the impact of early childhood education programs on children's school readiness, and effective methods for reducing classroom behavior problems and reducing the incidence of preschool expulsion. His scholarly writing addresses early childhood care and education programs, school readiness, and developmental assessment of young children. Dr. Gilliam actively provides consultation to state and federal decision makers.

His work has been covered in major national and international news outlets for print (e.g., *New York Times*, *Wall Street Journal*, *Washington Post*, *USA Today*, etc.), radio (e.g., *National Public Radio*), and television (e.g., *NBC Today Show*, *CBS The Early Show*, *ABC World News*, CNN, FOX, etc.).

Coti-Lynne Puamana Haia, JD, currently serves as the Bureau Chief for the Office of Hawaiian Affairs' Washington, D.C. Bureau. Born and raised on Oʻahu, Ms. Haia graduated from Gonzaga University in Spokane, Washington, with a bachelor's degree in political science. Upon graduating, Ms. Haia returned to Hawaiʻi to attend law school at the William S. Richardson School of Law. Ms. Haia worked briefly as a Deputy Prosecuting Attorney for the City and County of Honolulu before moving to Washington, D.C. to serve as a fellow in the office of U.S. Senator Daniel K. Inouye. She later moved to the office of U.S. Senator Mazie K. Hirono, eventually serving as Senator Hirono's Chief Counsel. She joined the Office of Hawaiian Affairs in 2016 and very much appreciates the opportunity to continue working for the State of Hawaiʻi and for the Native Hawaiian community.

Jeff Hutchinson, MD, FAAP, is a Colonel in the U.S. Army who has served since 1985 and graduated with a bachelor of science degree in chemistry from the United States Military Academy. He received a medical degree from the University of California San Francisco and completed a residency in pediatrics at Tripler Army Medical Center in Hawaii. He has served military families from Landstuhl, Germany, to Hawaiʻi and has cared for troops in task forces and other units. His specialty in adolescent medicine has allowed him to be an advocate of education and young adult health with publications in the *Journal of Pediatrics*, the *Journal of Military Medicine*, and the *Journal of Adolescent Health*. Currently, he is the Associate Dean of Clinical Affairs and Chief Diversity Officer for the F. Edward Hébert School of Medicine—"America's Medical School" Uniformed Services University. He serves on the National Academy of Medicine Board on Children Youth and Families and his research and national presentations focus on Media, Military Families, Education, Bias, and Sports Medicine.

Joseph Keaweʻaimoku Kaholokula, PhD, is an associate professor and Chair of Native Hawaiian Health in the John A. Burns School of Medicine at the University of Hawaiʻi at Mānoa. He is also a licensed clinical psychologist with a specialty in behavioral medicine. He received his PhD in clinical psychology from the University of Hawaiʻi at Mānoa in 2003 and completed a clinical health psychology postdoctoral fellowship in 2004 at the Triple Army Medical Center.

He has provided clinical services at various community health systems on Oʻahu and Maui in helping people to quit smoking, lose excess body weight, manage their hypertension and diabetes, and manage psychological factors that get in the way of people living healthy lives. He also provides training to other health care providers and community health advocates on topics relevant to culturally competent behavioral health services, motivational interviewing, behavioral strategies to health promotion, and Native Hawaiian and Pacific Islander health. He is a National Institutes of Health (NIH) funded researcher who examines how biological, behavioral, and social factors interplay to affect a person's risk for chronic diseases, such as diabetes and heart disease, especially in Asians, Native Hawaiians, and other Pacific Peoples. His research also involves developing sustainable, community-based health promotion programs to address obesity, diabetes, and heart disease disparities in Hawaiʻi for people of all ages.

Tracey Pérez Koehlmoos, PhD, MHA, serves as the Special Assistant to the Assistant Commandant of the Marine Corps. As senior program liaison for community health she serves as a senior representative of the Marine Corps on community health policy and research working groups at the interagency, Department of Defense, and Department of the Navy levels. As a recognized expert, she is tasked with making recommendations on complex issues requiring knowledge of administrative laws, policies, regulation, and precedent applicable to the administration of community health programs. Further, she monitors research to test new and best practices to improve the lives of marines, their families, and the communities in which they serve. Dr. Koehlmoos's research areas of interest led to the development of health service delivery for the home-less in Dhaka; scaling up zinc for the treatment of childhood diarrhea; and improving immunization services to children in hard-to-reach areas; as well as translation of evidence to policy with the Bangladesh Ministry of Health and Family Welfare and private sector organizations. She is an award-winning researcher and writer with more than 80 publications appearing in the *Lancet*, *PLoS Medicine*, the *Cochrane Library*, and *Health Policy* among others and a host of multimedia productions including television series and a documentary. A former Army Air Defense Artillery officer who earned the Army Commendation, Army Achievement, and Southwest Asia Service medals, Dr. Koehlmoos's post-Army awards include the Family Support Group Leader Europe Award, the Army Civilian Achievement Medal, and the Honorable Order of Joan d'Arc. She is a graduate of the Joint Military Attaché School. She is the widow of Colonel Randall Koehlmoos, US Army, and mother of Robert (USMA 2016), Michael, and David Koehlmoos.

Richard M. Lerner, PhD, is the Bergstrom Chair in Applied Developmental Science and the Director of the Institute for Applied Research in Youth Development at Tufts University. He went from kindergarten through PhD within the New York City public schools, completing his doctorate at the City University of New York in 1971 in developmental psychology. Lerner has more than 650 scholarly publications, including more than 75 authored or edited books. He was the founding editor of the *Journal of Research on Adolescence* and of *Applied Developmental Science*, which he continues to edit. Lerner is known for his theory of relations between life-span human development and social change, and for his research about the relations between adolescents and their peers, families, schools, and communities. As illustrated by his 2004 book, *Liberty: Thriving and Civic Engagement among America's Youth*, and his 2007 book, *The Good Teen: Rescuing Adolescence from the Myth of the Storm and Stress Years*, his work integrates the study of public policies and community-based programs with the promotion of positive youth development and youth contributions to civil society.

Nancy López, PhD, is associate professor of sociology at the University of New Mexico (BA Columbia College, Columbia University, 1991; PhD Graduate School & University Center, City University of New York [GSUC-CUNY], 1999). Dr. López directs and cofounded the Institute for the Study of "Race" and Social Justice, RWJF Center for Health Policy (race.unm.edu) and she is the founding coordinator of the New Mexico Statewide Race, Gender, Class Data Policy Consortium. Dr. López is also the inaugural cochair of the Diversity Council and serves on the Academic Freedom and Tenure Committee, UNM. Dr. López chairs the committee on the status of Racial and Ethnic Minorities and was past-chair of the Race, Gender, Class Section of the American Sociological Association. López's scholarship, teaching, and service is guided by the insights of intersectionality—the importance of examining race, gender, class, ethnicity together—for interrogating inequalities across a variety of social outcomes, including education, health, employment, housing, and developing contextualized solutions that advance social justice. Dr. López has taught for over two decades in a variety of public universities (City University of New York, University of Massachusetts, and University of New Mexico) that serve a very diverse group of students, including those who, like Dr. López, were the first in their families to complete high school and pursue higher education.

Raquel Mack, is a fifth-year doctoral candidate working toward a dual-track PhD in medical and clinical psychology at the Uniformed Services University of the Health Sciences (USUHS) in Bethesda, Maryland. While at USUHS Raquel has earned her MS in medical and clinical psychology, and completed a thesis on the effects of nicotine and stress on learning, memory, and information processing in an animal model. Raquel is currently working on her dissertation entitled "The effects of cultural competence and implicit bias on clinical decision making." Raquel attended Fisk University in Nashville, Tennessee, where she earned a BS (2010) in psychology, and Lipscomb University where she earned an MS (2012) in psychology. After college, Raquel was a Research Project Coordinator at Meharry Medical College (2011–2013) under the supervision of epidemiologist Dr. Maureen Sanderson working on several research projects with underserved populations including a provider intervention for human papillomavirus; an investigation of possible causes of breast cancer in African American breast cancer survivors; and a study of the relationships among hormones, diet, body size, and breast density in healthy African American and Hispanic women. Raquel's research interests include minority health disparities, implicit bias, and the effects of trauma on children in the juvenile justice system. Raquel's clinical interests include children and adolescents, community mental health, and psychodiagnostic assessment.

Jim Marks, MD, MPH, executive vice president, oversees all program, communications, research, and policy activities in support of the Robert Wood Johnson Foundation's vision to build a Culture of Health in America. Marks joined the Foundation in 2004 and was formerly the senior vice president and director of program portfolios. His areas of responsibility have included strengthening vulnerable families, healthy communities, transforming health and health care systems, achieving health equity, ensuring that all children grow up at a healthy weight, and New Jersey–focused programming.

Prior to joining RWJF, Marks served as assistant surgeon general and director of the Centers for Disease Control and Prevention's (CDC's) National Center for Chronic Disease Prevention and Health Promotion. Throughout his tenure at CDC, Marks developed and advanced systematic ways to prevent and detect diseases such as cancer, heart disease, and diabetes; reduce tobacco use; and address the nation's growing obesity epidemic.

A national leader in public health for more than 35 years, Marks has received numerous federal, state, and private awards from organizations such as the American Cancer Society, National Arthritis Foundation, Association of State and Territorial Health Officials, Council of State and Territorial Epidemiologists, Association of State and Territorial Chronic Disease Directors, and U.S. Public Health Service. He was elected to the Institute of Medicine of the National Academies in recognition of his accomplishments in epidemiology and public health. He has served on many governmental and nonprofit committees, including the Executive Board of the American Public Health Association. He is emeritus board chair of C-Change, whose members are the nation's key cancer leaders from government, business, and nonprofit sectors. He has published extensively in the areas of maternal and child health, health promotion, and chronic disease prevention.

Marks received an MD from the State University of New York at Buffalo. He trained as a pediatrician at the University of California at San Francisco, and was a Robert Wood Johnson Clinical Scholar at Yale University, where he received his MPH.

Shantel E. Meek, PhD, serves as a Policy Advisor for Early Childhood Development in the Administration for Children and Families at the U.S. Department of Health and Human Services (HHS). In her role, Dr. Meek advises the Deputy Assistant Secretary for Early Childhood Development on a wide array of research areas and policy issues, including parent and community engagement, promoting healthy child development, and supporting young children with disabilities. Prior to her work at HHS, Dr. Meek served as a Clinical Interventionist for children with autism spectrum disorder (ASD) and their families at the Southwest Autism Research and Resource Center (SARRC). In this capacity, she worked one-on-one with children, performed educational consultation and inclusion support services, and trained parents and paraprofessionals on empirically supported techniques aimed at improving social, emotional, cognitive, motor, and self-help skills in young children with ASD. Dr. Meek's research activities are focused on the healthy social-emotional and cognitive development of young children in poverty and young children with developmental disabilities. Dr. Meek's work related to the social development of children with ASD has been published in peer-reviewed journals. She holds a BA in psychology and a PhD in family and human development from Arizona State University.

Noreen Mokuau, DSW, is Dean and Professor at the Myron B. Thompson School of Social Work at the University of Hawai'i at Mānoa. As a Native Hawaiian woman, she is committed to social work education that is anchored in excellence and founded in the unique attributes of Hawai'i and the Pacific-Asia region. She is a graduate of the Kamehameha Schools, the University of Hawai'i Mānoa (BA psychology; MSW social work) and the University of California, Los Angeles (DSW social welfare). She received the UH Regents Excellence in Teaching Award and the UH Community Service Award.

Presently, she is Coprincipal Investigator and Director of Hā Kūpuna: National Resource Center for Native Hawaiian Elders, and serves as a Commissioner on the Council on Social Work Education Commission for Diversity and Social and Economic Justice. Dr. Mokuau has edited three books, published numerous journal articles, book chapters, and technical reports, and given many presentations on cultural competency and social services for Native Hawaiians, Pacific Islanders, and Asian Americans.

As a scholar, mentor, and teacher, Mokuau's interests in cultural competency centers on social justice issues, including health disparities among Native Hawaiian, Pacific Islander, and Asian populations, and caregiving issues for culturally diverse elders. A strong advocate for community-based participatory research, her research is rooted in the 'ohana and community. She acknowledges that her life work is based on the direction and guidance of her own 'ohana, with special credit to the legacy of her parents.

Velma McBride Murry, PhD, is the Lois Autrey Betts Chair in Education and Human Development and Professor, Human and Organizational Development in Peabody College at Vanderbilt University. Her work has focused on the significance of context in studies of African American families and youth, particularly the impact of racism on family functioning. This research has elucidated the dynamics of this contextual stressor in the everyday life of African Americans and the ways family members buffer each other from the impact of the external stressors that cascade through African American lives. Professor McBride Murry served as principal investigator of The Strong African American Families Program, a universal RCT prevention trial designed to deter HIV-related risk behavior among rural African American youth residing in Georgia. Murry received continued support from NIMH to conduct a RCT in Tennessee to determine the efficacy and viability of a technology-driven, interactive, family-based preventive intervention, the Pathways for African American Success Program, as a delivery modality for rural families.

Ken Peake, DSW, is Chief Operating Officer and Assistant Director, Mount Sinai Adolescent Health Center (MSAHC) in New York City. Dr. Peake was MSAHC's Director of Mental Health from 1990 until 2002 and is an assistant professor in the Icahn School of Medicine at Mount Sinai. He has his master's degree in social work from Hunter College and his doctorate in social welfare from the Graduate Center at the City University of New York. Dr. Peake has numerous peer-reviewed publications and book chapters related to the well-being of inner-city adolescents and to reducing trauma in this population. He believes that to serve young people well we must develop smart organizations with a "reflective" organizational culture that encourages innovation. Born in Wales, Dr. Peake trained as an architect and fell into his current career in 1973 as a youth worker on Manhattan's Lower East. For a decade he worked with homeless families and with children of abused women using a combination of the arts, counseling, and family therapy approaches to engage young people and their families. He then spent another decade as a practitioner in community-based mental health, and in private psychotherapy practice.

Dwayne Proctor, PhD, senior adviser to the President and director, believes that the Foundation's vision for building a Culture of Health presents a unique opportunity to achieve health equity by advancing and promoting innovative systems changes related to the social determinants of health.

Proctor came to the Robert Wood Johnson Foundation (RWJF) in 2002 as a senior communications and program officer, providing strategic guidance and resources for several child health and risk-prevention initiatives like the Nurse-Family Partnership, Free to Grow, Leadership to Keep Children Alcohol-Free, Partnership for a Drug-Free America and the National Campaign to Prevent Teenage Pregnancy. In 2005, Proctor was tapped to lead RWJF's national strategies to reverse the rise in childhood obesity rates. In this role, he worked with his colleagues to (1) promote effective changes to public policies and industry practices; (2) test and demonstrate innovative community and school-based environmental changes; and (3) use both "grassroots" and "treetops" advocacy approaches to educate leaders on their roles in preventing childhood obesity. Proctor is known for his strategic collaborations, having worked on several cross-sector initiatives (e.g., Partnership for a Healthier America, the evaluation of the Healthy Weight Commitment Foundation, ChildObesity 180) and national programs that focused on decreasing childhood obesity disparities gaps (e.g., Healthy Schools Program; Salud America!; Healthy Kids, Healthy Communities; Communities Creating Healthy Environments; National Policy and Legal Action Network; and Voices for Healthy Kids). In 2014, as multiple municipalities and states were reporting signs of progress in reversing the childhood obesity epidemic, Proctor was reassigned to direct RWJF's work to eliminate health disparities.

Before coming to the Foundation, Proctor was an assistant professor at the University of Connecticut School of Medicine where he taught courses on health communication and marketing to multicultural populations. During his Fulbright Fellowship in Senegal, West Africa, his research team investigated how HIV/AIDS prevention messages raised awareness of AIDS as a national health problem. Proctor received his doctoral, master's and bachelor's degrees in marketing and communication science from the University of Connecticut. He is the former chairman of the board of directors for the Association of Black Foundation Executives and currently is the chairman of the board of trustees for the National Association for the Advancement of Colored People.

Srividya Ramasubramanian, PhD, MA, is Associate Dean for Climate & Inclusion in the College of Liberal Arts and Associate Professor of Communication at Texas A&M University. She is Cofounder and Executive Director of Media Rise, a global alliance for media educators, creative media professionals, activists, and artists committed to media for social good with over 3,000 members. Ramasubramanian specializes in media psychology, gender and racial stereotyping, global media and social change, and cultural diversity. Her research primarily looks at how media stereotypes and counter-stereotypes influence audiences' attitudes about race, gender, nationality, and sexuality. Her recent projects examine implicit racial/gender stereotypes, prejudice reduction, digital new media literacy, and mindfulness media. She has published in leading journals such as *Communication Research*, *Communication Monographs*, *Media Psychology*, *Sex Roles*, and *Journal of Social Issues*. Her work has been featured in the *Huffington Post*, *National Public Radio*, *Dallas Morning News*, and *India Today* apart from local media outlets. She has delivered several public talks and keynotes including at the London School of Economics, National University of Singapore, V University of Amsterdam, Hanover University, and the Communication University of China. She is/was editorial board member of journals such as *Communication Monographs*, *Journal of International & Intercultural Communication*, and *Journal of Applied Communication Research*.

Robert Seidel, MLA, is an adjunct faculty member in philosophy at McDaniel College in Westminster, Maryland, focusing on political philosophy. He cofacilitates two undergraduate seminars, "Changing the World: Philosophical Theory and Policy Practice" and "Violence/Nonviolence: Ends, Means, and Political Philosophy." He is also an independent consultant in Baltimore, focusing on education and youth development practice, policy, and advocacy. Prior to launching his consulting practice in 2014, Bob was Senior Director, Strategic Initiatives and Policy, for the National Summer Learning Association, where he worked on federal and state policy, strategic partnerships, and community-systems-building initiatives. He also spent a decade in the national office of Communities In Schools, serving as National Program Partnership Director and Government Resources Director, among other roles. Bob's professional work has included being a teacher in the Baltimore City Public Schools, an administrator and faculty member at the Johns Hopkins University Institute for Policy Studies, and Service-Learning Specialist at the federal Corporation for National and Community Service. He holds a bachelor of arts degree in sociology with honors and distinction from the University of Michigan as well as a master of liberal arts degree from Johns Hopkins University.

Sadé Soares is a rising, fourth-year clinical psychology graduate student at the Uniformed Services University of the Health Sciences (USUHS). She graduated from the United States Military Academy at West Point with a bachelor of science in psychology. Sadé is an Army Captain with nine years of active duty service. Prior to attending graduate school, she held several military leadership positions which included leading peers, enlisted members, and civilian government employees. Since beginning at USUHS, Sadé has served as an interventionist on studies aimed at preventing obesity and fostering healthy lifestyle changes. As a student, she has experienced much joy and growth working as a clinical teaching assistant and providing peer supervision. Sadé's clinical interests include child and family problems, trauma, and psychosocial difficulties due to cultural factors. Her research interests include the intersectionality of historical trauma, cultural affiliation, and health factors. Currently, Sadé serves as the Student Chair of the District of Columbia Psychological Association. Sadé spends her free time playing with her infant son and taking on the world with her husband.

Patrick H. Tolan, PhD, is a professor at the University of Virginia in the Curry School of Education and in the Department of Psychiatry and Neurobehavioral Sciences in the School of Medicine. He is director of the cross-university multidisciplinary center, Youth-Nex: The U.Va. Center to Promote Effective Youth Development. Established in 2009, Youth-Nex is a transdisciplinary nexus, focusing on the capabilities of young people in connection to health, communities, schools, and relationships engaging over 30 faculty across grounds. He leads the center's mission to promote healthy youth development, to enhance the potential of youth as productive citizens and to reduce developmental risk, through focused research, training, and service. Youth-Nex collaborates at the local, state, and national levels to help apply innovations and best practices and engages in international collaborations on measuring and promoting youth development. It is now recognized nationally as a leading voice in research for direction in optimizing development of our children. Over the past 30 years Professor Tolan has conducted many research studies on youth development, programs to affect youth development and prevent problems, and to understand and affect youth violence.

Sharon Toomer Sharon Toomer is the recently appointed Executive Director of the National Association of Black Journalists (NABJ). Sharon has an extensive background in public affairs, communications, journalism and new media. Prior to joining NABJ, she served as the Senior Vice President, Public Affairs & Policy at a public relations agency, and as the Chief of Staff & Senior Policy

Advisor for U.S. Representative (D.C.-Shadow) Franklin Garcia. Sharon is also the founder of the award-winning digital news and information publication, BlackandBrownNews.com (BBN), where she was inspired to develop her perspective on community violence. She is the past recipient of the CUNY Graduate School of Journalism Political Reporting Fellowship, and her wide-range of experiences and multicultural worldview has earned her awards in journalism excellence, and appearances on television, radio, print and digital news outlets. Sharon lives in the Washington, D.C. area, and is a proud alumna of Spelman College.

JoAnn U. Tsark, MPH, is a Public Health Educator based in Hawai'i, where she has spent more than three decades working to reduce health disparities experienced by Native Hawaiian and Pacific Islanders. She currently is Research Director of Papa Ola Lokahi (Native Hawaiian Board of Health), Program Director for 'Imi Hale–Native Hawaiian Cancer Network (funded since 2000; U01CA86105/U01CA114630/U54CA153459), Colead of the Community-Based Research Core for the RCMI Multidisciplinary and Translational Research Infrastructure (RMATRIX, 2U54MD007584-04) at the UH Medical School, and instructor at the UH Office of Public Health Studies. In these roles, she has been instrumental in developing a robust, community-based infrastructure to increase community-based, participatory research (CBPR) that focuses on community-identified priorities. She founded Hawai'i's first community-based IRB, established an evidence-based cancer patient navigation training program, developed more than 100 culturally tailored education materials, and provided CBPR training and mentorship to hundreds of Native Hawaiians, Pacific Islanders, and students interested in indigenous health. Ms. Tsark has developed and maintains an extensive network of local, national, and international community and academic partners to support Papa Ola Lokahi's work in the prevention and control of diabetes, cardiovascular risk disease, and cancer in Native Hawaiian and Pacific Islander communities.

Alford A. Young Jr., PhD, is the Arthur F. Thurnau Professor and Chair of the Department of Sociology at the University of Michigan. Professor Young has pursued research on low-income, urban-based African Americans, employees at an automobile manufacturing plant, African American scholars and intellectuals, and the classroom-based experiences of higher-education faculty as they pertain to diversity and multiculturalism. He employs ethnographic interviewing as his primary data collection method. His principal scholarly objective has been to explore how the social experiences of African Americans shape the emergence of what sociologist Erving Goffman referred to as schemata of interpretation. These schemata include worldviews, belief systems, and ideologies. Here his work has centered on exploring the connections between the social location of individuals (i.e., differences in types of residential experiences, work histories, schooling experiences, etc.) and the content of their worldviews and beliefs systems about mobility, the world of work, and other social issues and conditions. His objective in research on low-income African American men, his primary area of research, has been to argue for a renewed cultural sociology of the African American urban poor. Essentially, he argues that behavior is not solely produced and regulated by values and norms, but is also affected by the beliefs, worldviews, and personal ideologies that people construct, adapt, and/or employ in forming what are, for them, common-sense understandings of social reality. More specifically, he explores how those understandings emerge in different form based on individuals' patterns of social exposure to people who are positioned differently in various social hierarchies (racial, ethnic, class based, etc.).

CPSIA information can be obtained
at www.ICGtesting.com
Printed in the USA
LVHW071656050822
725273LV00026B/1724